# The Secret Habits of Happy Humans

**Allen Young**

First  published 2007.

ISBN   **978-1-84753-584-9**

# Contents

# Chapter 1

# Introduction

## Sections in Chapter 1

# Chapter 1

# Contentment

## 1.1  Introduction

The title promises that people who are generally happy have identifiable common habits.  It also suggests that they are not well-known or obvious – so we call them "secret habits".  So if this is true, and we can identify the secret habits, there must be something that we can do about our state of contentment.  And there is.  This book will explain the common factors that are found in people who experience a positive sense of contentment, and will lead you through explanations and exercises where you can check how you compare.

Some people achieve their state of happiness without having consciously worked their way through the issues.  They are fortunate.  Most of us need to apply thought and energy to the process before we achieve or realise our happiness.

A fundamental wish for most people is to be a "contented" human being. In fact you have probably noticed that it is only those who have achieved this foundation who can move on to be a truly effective leader, manager, father, mother, daughter or son, or whatever they aspire to be. Other achievements in life can seem empty unless we achieve a feeling of contentment. As a result of searching for the wrong thing, many of us set ourselves an endless series of goals and targets without ever feeling truly content.

This book will take you through an explanation of six key factors that are crucial to the achievement of contentment. It will also show you how to analyse your own current state. Think of the process as your "Contentment Project". There are short questionnaires to complete, and guided exercises to follow, which will allow you to identify what you can do to achieve a greater feeling of contentment. When you have finished the book you will have made significant progress on your Contentment Project, and you will have an action plan specifically for your situation.

But first a bit of history and explanation. It is important to be clear about what we mean by contentment, and there are important lessons from the theories and studies that already exist.

## Money.

Most people will agree with propositions about the inability of money to make us happy. Our behaviour often shows that we haven't totally accepted the proposition, but intellectually at least most people accept it. Herzberg and Maslow have been popular reading with their propositions of Hygiene factors, Motivators, and in Maslow's case the Hierarchy of Needs. His hierarchy ranges from basic physiological drives to self esteem, and at the top of his list "self-actualisation". Most people seem to accept all of it intellectually and can discuss the inability of material wealth or possessions to provide what we usually call "true happiness".  But we mostly continue to seek these supposedly impotent goals.

However as human beings we are capable of holding contradictory views at the one time.  Picture yourself travelling in the peaceful countryside, coming across an old farmer leaning on a gate and quietly smoking his pipe. Who can resist the thought "now there is a happy man"?  Similarly when on holiday in a remote Mediterranean village, most people who see a picturesque fisherman at work on his nets experience at least some feeling of envy for the apparent happiness of the individual.  It seems such a striking contrast to our complicated, over-busy, driven lives.  We long for an unspecified simple contentment.  But most of us continue to behave as if material success will bring the contentment we are looking for.

This introduction will explain what I mean by the phrase "contented human being", drawing not only on professional experience, but also on the writings of philosophers and psychologists who have examined the idea.  The book then details a widely applicable set of six factors that can be used as indicators and benchmarks. Crucially they also provide a basis for planning some action.

What makes this approach different from many others is the holistic view which suggests that one can only achieve the component parts within a satisfactory "whole".

When you have finished reading this book, I hope you will have found yourself thinking more deeply about what really matters to you, and on the basis of that, measured yourself in your own terms.  And finally I hope that the framework will have given you a practical basis for planning some action, and the achievement of a greater level of contentment.

## 1.2    The Contented Human Being

What is important to me?   When I think about this I almost inevitably start thinking of the themes in my life, and depending on my mood and circumstance I may focus on the context of my role as father or as son, or at other times on my job as director or colleague.   You may focus on all sorts of roles that apply to you.   These are what we mean by the "themes" in your life.   You can probably identify 7 or 8 themes that are most important to you. But have you ever experienced them as completely separate aspects of life? Is it possible to excel in one, fail in others, and feel contentment?

Our proposition is that whatever the career or walk of life, more pervasive, more fundamental than "success" in any one dimension is a deeper feeling of contentment.   They are not mutually exclusive concepts. Think of the underlying contentment as a solid foundation that can help us cope with the ups and downs of the different aspects of life.   There may be aspects of life that are not exactly as we would wish just at the moment, but they need not completely disable the rest of our well-being.   Achieving the solid foundation helps in all the other aspects of life, and helps us maintain the balance necessary for clear thinking and good judgement.

It is perfectly possible to be enormously successful in some themes in life and still not achieve the elusive feeling of contentment.   We can probably think of fortunate individuals who are enormously successful in some field, whether artistic, commercial, or sporting, who also seem to exude the contentment of being at peace with themselves.   However we all have also seen or listened to highly successful men and women, who exude the opposite.   They demonstrate a grating discontent with themselves which usually spills over into the unpleasant way they relate to and treat other people. It would be unkind to name them - you can make your own list! There is a little diagram that is relevant:

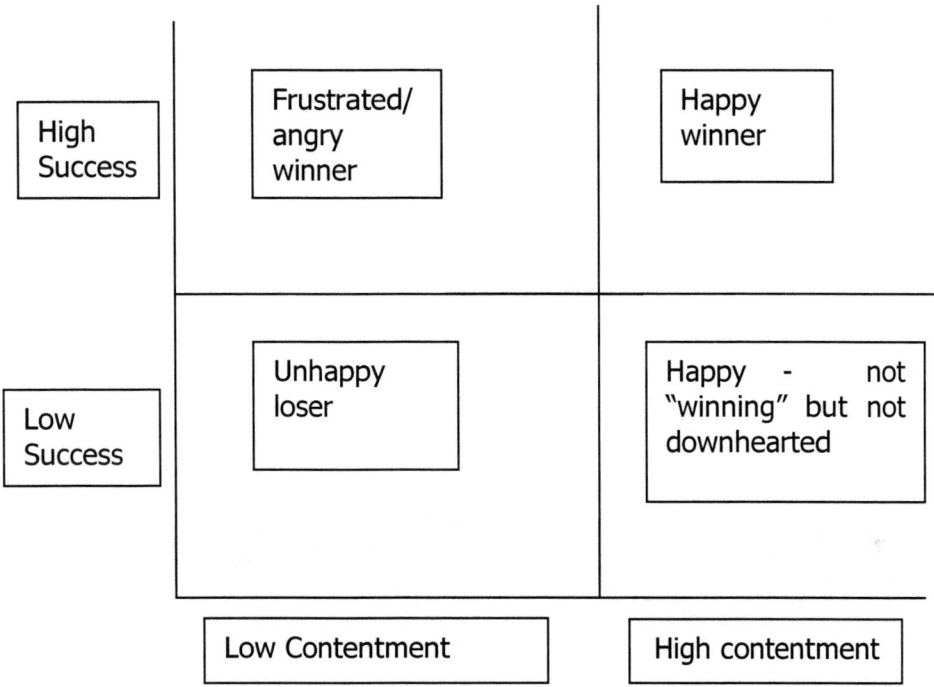

We will explore the way this works in more detail, but in the meantime a quote from the playwright August Strindberg. His life has been described as one of "restless ambition and constant conflict". In an interview in 1897 he declared that anyone's greatest potential misfortune was "to lack inner peace and a quiet conscience."

## 1.3    Ideas of contentment

"Contentment" is a broad concept, and we link many other behaviours, attitudes and responses to it.  For example if you imagine the person who embodies each of the following descriptions, you are likely to make the judgement that the individual is to a large extent a contented human being.

- The contented human being - at peace with themselves

- The happy human - not just passively content, but consciously and positively happy

- The considerate friend - showing consideration for others and enjoying positive relationships

- The balanced individual - who is not at the mercy of any one aspect of themselves

- The rational being - who isn't likely to persist with irrational thoughts and actions

- The moral human - who acts in accordance with a set of moral principles

The Greeks had an interesting insight into the issue. Aristotle, Plato and Socrates all used the term "Eudaemonia" – which can be loosely translated as a "good spirit within". What is interesting about their writings is that they were very clear that this was tied up with their view of the virtuous life. Happiness for them was tied up with Values, and the contented human needed to be an honourable human. Lasting happiness was very clearly seen as something that was not achievable by the "unjust".

The Greeks also had views that are extremely relevant to us today about the necessity of having a **vision** of how one can be. They believed that true happiness was achievable only in pursuit and achievement of a virtuous vision for life. They believed in the necessity of a balance between our human desires hungers and ambitions, and the extent to which they are satisfied. That probably doesn't surprise anyone, but the combination of the ideas provides an important thread that will emerge throughout the book.


## 1.4   Mood, state, or condition?

Studies of happiness and contentment usually identify three or four different meanings of the word "happiness".

- First of all there is the reactive feeling of happiness about something specific – for example you might be happy with a gift you receive that briefly lifts your mood.

- Secondly there is the temporary mood where we feel generally positive, optimistic or happy for no identifiable reason. This is usually a short term experience.

- Thirdly there is personality tendency towards a sunny disposition – something most likely inherited and a life-long bonus.

- Fourthly there is the state of happiness and contentment in life, which is more long-lasting and pervasive than the reaction or temporary mood, and is more firmly based and conscious than the simple cheerful disposition. It is this fourth fundamental state that is the concern of this book.

## 1.5 Does it make any difference?

How can I ask such a question!  Some of you will say of course it makes a difference – I wouldn't be reading the book if I didn't believe that it is important to achieve a feeling of contentment.  That doesn't necessarily prove that it makes a difference.  We can feel that all sorts of things are important and worth putting money and energy into achieving, only to be left with an empty feeling of dissatisfaction in the end.  So is "contentment" just another false goal?

Interestingly the Harvard academic George Valliant conducted a series of long-term studies which are relevant to the question.  He has described one long-term study of a group of students which followed them from college in the 1940s through to old age.  Among many fascinating threads of information, he found positive correlations between life-satisfaction (or contentment) and longevity, along with lower likelihood of serious physical or mental illness.  His long term study found that contentment was not connected with wealth or specific job seniority, but it was directly connected to happiness with their work.  It was also related to a balanced life, indicated by a greater ability to take the holidays they were entitled to.  Yes it is true, those of us who are too driven to be able to take time for holidays are likely to be less well and less happy than those who are able to take the time.

So contentment is desirable not just because it is a pleasurable state. It is desirable because it is better for our mental and physical health.  I doubt if that is any surprise to you.

## 1.6    The essential components for human contentment:

The essential components for contentment need to satisfy a number of tests.  The six used in this book have been checked to make sure they make sense against a synthesis of the ideas already quoted, which come from philosophers ancient and modern.  They also have been checked against the findings from academic studies of happiness and contentment.  And they have been based on observation and listening to a great variety of individuals in many years of counselling and coaching.  These are the underpinning foundations for the descriptions of the "contented human being".

- A concept of "who you are" that includes realistic perceptions of your strengths, weaknesses, preferences and dislikes,

- A set of beliefs or Values that provide a moral framework you can articulate, refer to, and which guide your decisions, standards and behaviours,

- A set of "drivers" or goals that you have been able to choose for yourself that give you purpose and energy,

- Satisfying relationships with others,

- The resources you need to allow you some achievement of your chosen goals.

- Some record of achievement that leads to a realistic and positive self-confidence.

The rest of the book is divided into six main sections, each one describing the factor, giving some explanatory examples and providing a self-assessment checklist.

The final section is devoted to pulling together all the self assessment you have carried out and giving a usable method of keeping your plans and progress under review.

You will find that there are worksheets in every chapter that encourage you to engage in some guided self analysis. These are carefully structured to draw on real evidence. Where possible you will not simply be asked for your opinion about yourself on the relevant factor. You will be enabled to answer some questions that gather evidence about "what actually happens", or "what I did each evening this week". The worksheets will help you to keep your analysis real, practical, and based on evidence.

# Chapter 2

## Who I am

### Sections in Chapter 2

**2.1**     **Clear picture of who I am**

**2.2**     **Taking stock**

**2.3**     **History**

**2.4**     **Strengths**

**2.5**     **Preferences**

**2.6**     **Dark side**

**2.7**     **Ongoing self-review**

# Chapter 2

## 2.1  Clear picture of who I am....

Most people when asked to describe themselves are completely stumped. We generally have neither the practice, the "headings", nor the words to use to describe ourselves.  The summaries we write in our CVs rarely seem to capture us – they can seem to be a separate and slightly embarrassing paper description that would not be the complete answer to this truly fundamental question.

This chapter will describe several different ways of getting to grips with the question.  It will give examples of how people have used them and will give you some practical worksheets to use.

The headings that you will work through are:


- Taking stock – the idea and value of taking stock of who you are and what are your key attributes.
- History – how to use your history to be clearer about who you are
- Strengths – making a realistic inventory of a wide variety of potential strengths
- Preferences – being clear about your natural preferences and how they make you different from everyone else.
- Dark side – facing up to the things you are not so good at, and the situations that do not suit you
- Ongoing self-review – how to keep a realistic and up-to-date self-assessment.

## 2.2　Taking stock.

The term may conjure up pictures of dusty old shops and stores, and equally dusty old clerks with checklists adding up items on shelves. Don't let it put you off. Taking stock of yourself and your world is the first step to being able to manage your way successfully through it. Think of it like any other project, whether cooking a meal, assembling a piece of furniture, or packing for a holiday. You need to know what you have so that you can spot the gaps, and it's wise to make sure you have the bits you need before starting to cook, build or pack, never mind manage your future.

Taking stock is crucial not only in order to enable you to move forward, but also as an important part of your "contentment project". You may find that you have greater riches than you realised whether in terms of strengths, achievements or relationships. There is no point in putting energy into fixing something that is already well provided while ignoring the area that is lacking.

When you walk into someone else's house it is easier for you to spot the little things that need attention than it is for the householder to spot them. Similarly at work, we can focus on the things we are in the habit of focussing on, until either someone else helps us see what is missing, or we undertake a systematic and objective review of what we do and how we do it. Observe yourself at work or at home, your manager at work, your subordinates and your colleagues. There is a strong human tendency to do the things that either come easily, or that we have learned to derive satisfaction from. Jobs are adjusted slightly to suit the jobholder's preferences. Things that get done around the house are the things that someone has learned a way of doing – but they aren't necessarily the right things or all the things needing attention.

The same principle applies to the way we organise our lives. Unless we stand back and take a structured look at ourselves we are at the mercy of three things:

1. Our habits – the way we have become used to behaving – whether it is doing the same sort of things again, or at the other extreme a habit of relentless change.
2. What happens – unless we have our own set of priorities we have no way of resisting the moment to moment and day to day pressures that life hits us with.
3. Other people – who can be either thoughtless or worse, calculating, and may make use of us to suit their plans and priorities.

So the process of taking stock is your starting point for managing your way through the project, and a necessary foundation for the subsequent thinking and planning you will undertake.

## 2.3    History.

"*The hasty reformer who does not remember the past will find himself condemned to repeat it.*" John Buchan

Each of us has a wealth of information about ourselves stored in our memories.  Unfortunately we rarely access it in a structured way so that we can make the best use of what we can learn from it.  Some people repress the unpleasant memories that remind them of difficult times.  Some people do the opposite, and are so wrapped up in the bad times that they find it difficult to focus on the positives.  Neither approach is useful in learning from past experiences.

*Brian is a middle-aged professional, with many typical professional tendencies.  He is well-organised, something of a perfectionist, and takes very good care of his possessions – some might say too much care.  He suffered what might be termed a cautious mid-life crisis.  He had the crisis but didn't take off for South America on a motorbike, or leave his wife and children.  However he sank into a serious depression in which every aspect of his life seemed unsatisfactory.  In particular, he became disillusioned about his marriage and wrestled with the possibility of making a fresh start with another partner.  He also came to feel that his work was unsuccessful and unfulfilling, which also left him on the verge of deciding to make a dramatic change.*

*A series of life review sessions helped him to chart the good times and the bad times in his adult life.  A pattern emerged that he had been unaware of.  He learned that in his personal life, a lot of the good times were*

associated with new experiences. Many of his "highs" were when he had tried a new sport, explored a new holiday destination, or discovered a new friendship. Significantly, many of those "highs" had been shared with his partner.

Similarly in his professional life, the highs almost always were associated with change, and with new challenges. He was actually able to catalogue many successes when forced to look back systematically and own up to his successes rather than remembering the failures.

He had failed to realise the extent to which variety was important to him. And he had missed the data that was in his memory that showed how he had in the past achieved very satisfying variety with his existing partner and in his existing career. He was able to create a set of plans which would inject the missing variety into both his professional and private lives. A new project in his professional work fired him with renewed enthusiasm, and within months he could scarcely believe that he had contemplated giving it up. A new enthusiasm for exploring the Far East with his wife led to new shared experiences and a new lease of life for their partnership.

## Your history line:

Use the chart below or make a large scale chart on which to chart your highs, lows and in-betweens. The y axis represents your feelings – enormously simplified. The higher the line the better you were feeling at the time. The x axis represents time. You can choose the time period, but it is best to make it most or all of your adult life.

(You may find it better to use a large separate piece of paper for this.)

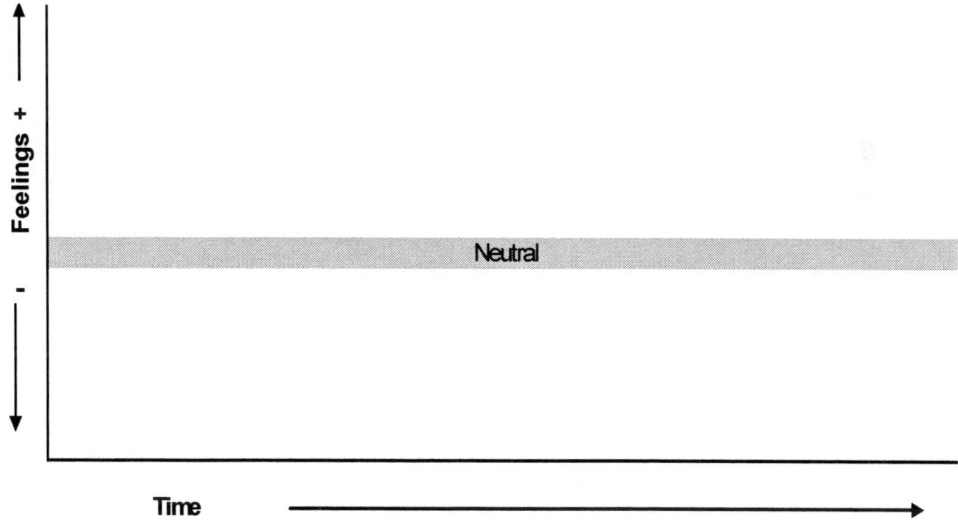

1. Label the time-line with dates and mark memorable events. Then take your time and draw the line that gives you a graphical representation of the highs and lows of your feelings.

2. Think back over each of the highs. Make notes of how you felt; what in retrospect made you feel that way; what were the significant features of the time; and what you can learn from the recollection.

3. Think back over each of the lows.  Make notes similar to those on the highs.

4. What have you learned from your history?  Make a few notes of key points to factor in to the later work you will do.

## 2.4   Strengths

You may have found that the history-line exercise has already helped you think of some of your strengths.  This needs to be taken a step further, and once again you will need a structure to help you think systematically and to avoid the self-imposed modesty or unconscious blind-spots that most people live with.

The headings we are going to use are simple and you can add to them if you like.  You will find a work-sheet in this chapter that you can use for your notes.

- Mental strengths
- Physical
- Emotional
- People
- Organisational

First of all an exercise.  Take the worksheet labelled Evidence of Strengths. Your task is to think back over the occasions when:-

- Someone has asked <u>you</u> specifically to help
- You have done something which you know was a satisfying "job-well-done"
- Someone has told you that you were missed because you would have done something differently
- You are routinely asked to carry out a particular role
- You have a strong feeling that you could have done something better than the person you have watched.

In one column note briefly the occasion or comment. In the other note the conclusion you can reach about either your strengths or about the image others have of you.

**Evidence of Strengths: (Sample)**

| Piece of evidence | Strength |
|---|---|
| • Someone e-mails to say they missed me from the conference – they mention the atmosphere and my humour | People must see me as contributing positively to the humour and to the good atmosphere of meetings! |
| • June asks me about how to deal with tricky issue of her tax | Knowledgeable and sensible? |
| • Membership committee asks me to continue as secretary | Organised and good with written material? |
| • Neighbour asks me about computer issue | IT literate and competent. |
| • I'm always asked in a group what wine we should have | Reputation for wine knowledge and good judgement! |
| • My frustration at badly chaired meeting yesterday – I know I do better than that | Chairing meetings |
| • Friend asks me to help with choosing finance deal for new car | Practical, knowledgeable, sensible. |

As you work your way through a list of simple things that happen, you need to set your modesty aside and ask yourself what that says about you. If you are frequently asked to help friends or colleagues with computer issues – that tells you something. Be honest and positive about your self-assessment.

## Evidence of Strengths

| Piece of evidence | Strength |
|---|---|
| • | |
| • | |
| • | |
| • | |
| • | |
| • | |
| • | |
| • | |

The next step is to use the strengths you have identified along with those you can straightforwardly identify for yourself, and to slot them into the categories in the worksheets. The divisions we are using are:

- Mental – to list all those things related to the knowledge you have, or the thinking and judgement you are able to demonstrate

- Physical – to identify the more physical skills and aptitudes you can claim, whether they are learned skills, or simply a general ability

- Emotional – to list the ways in which your emotions are helpful, whether in terms of balance, restraint, or as a driver

- People – many of the mental and emotional strengths will be particularly relevant to how you relate to other people. This is such an important area that it has its own heading.

- Organisational – similarly strengths you have already identified may have particular relevance in organising things. But this is another important area worthy of its own heading, even though you may end up with some repetition of other strengths.

The following pages are set out as worksheets with some prompt words and questions. Take your time to work through them. You may not be able to do it all in one session. Take a few days with the sheets available, or transfer the headings into your PDA or notebook so that you can record ideas as you have them.

*There is a page on each category, then a highlighting exercise which creates your list of "essential me" strengths, and provides some data for the later planning work.*

**Mental** –  list all those things related to the knowledge you have, or the thinking and judgement you are able to demonstrate:  (Don't feel bound by the prompt words!)

| *Domain* | *Strength   (prompts are suggestions and not exclusive)* | *Important?* <br> *Tick key strengths* |
|---|---|---|
| **Knowledge** | Technical? <br><br> Language? <br><br> Geographical? <br><br> Professional? <br><br> Sport-related? <br><br> Financial? <br><br> Others? | |
| **Thinking** | Intelligence? <br><br>        Words?  Numbers?  Practical? <br><br> Analysis? <br><br> Memory? <br><br> Complexity? <br><br> Clarity? | |
| **Judgement** | Wisdom? <br><br> Balance? <br><br> Decisiveness? <br><br> Compassion? <br><br> Coping with ambiguity/ missing data? | |

**Physical** – identify the physical skills and aptitudes you can claim, whether they are learned skills, or a general ability

| *Domain* | *Strength* | *Important?* <br> *Tick key strengths* |
|---|---|---|
| **Aptitude** | Co-ordination hand/eye? <br><br> Reactions? <br><br> Physical movement? <br><br> Graphical? <br><br> Musical? | |
| **Developed skills** | Sporting skill? <br><br> DIY/Tool-handling? <br><br> Painting/drawing? <br><br> Playing instrument? <br><br> Gardening? <br><br> Driving? | |
| **General** | Physical strength/fitness? <br><br> Walking/running? | |

**Emotional** –   list the ways in which your emotions are helpful, whether in terms of balance, restraint, or as a driver

| *Domain* | *Strength* | *Important?*<br>*Tick key strengths* |
|---|---|---|
| **Empathy** | Able to understand others?<br>Able to deal with distress?<br>Patience?<br>Interest? | |
| **Stability/ Volatility** | Self-confidence?<br>Able to cope with stress?<br>Know when to "Blow"?<br>Confidence to stand up for principle?<br>Dealing with uncertainty? | |
| **Self-regulation** | Strong set of guidelines?<br>Consistent reactions?<br>Coherent behaviour? | |

To help think about this page you may like to think about the situations or issues that you don't deal with as well as you would like, as well as those you are comfortable with.

**People** – many of the mental and emotional strengths will be particularly relevant to how you relate to other people.  This is such an important area that it has its own heading.

| *Domain* | *Strength* | *Important?* <br> *Tick key strengths* |
|---|---|---|
| **Relating** | Able to create positive relationships? <br><br> Listening? <br><br> Being understood? <br><br> Communicating effectively? <br><br> One-to-one? <br><br> Group relations? | |
| **Supporting** | Making contact? <br><br> Keeping in touch? <br><br> Giving feedback? <br><br> Helping with problems? | |
| **Confronting** | Honest feedback? <br><br> Seeing other side? <br><br> Challenging views? <br><br> Disagreeing? | |

**Organisational** – strengths you have already identified may have particular relevance in organising things – this applies not necessarily to work but equally to home, or to any of your activities.

| *Domain* | *Strength* | *Important?*<br>*Tick key strengths* |
|---|---|---|
| **Strategy and planning** | *Thinking strategically?*<br>*Explaining issues clearly?*<br>*Avoiding losing the plot?* | |
| **Operational** | *Budgets?*<br>*Managing money?*<br>*Planning meetings?*<br>*Chairing?*<br>*Involving people?*<br>*Administration?*<br>*Getting things done?* | |
| **IT/Paper** | *Writing?*<br>*Drafting for others?*<br>*Recording?*<br>*Research?* | |

## Summary of strengths:

*From the preceding pages select the strengths that fit into the following categories:*

| | Strength | Action?<br>(tick if YES) |
|---|---|---|
| Strengths that I have that I am most pleased to have. | •<br>•<br>•<br>•<br>• | |
| Strengths that I have that are not important to me. | •<br>• | |
| Strengths that I DO NOT have that I would <u>like to</u> have. | •<br>•<br>•<br>• | |
| Strengths that I DO NOT have that I am clear I do not have and am unlikely ever to have. (And that's OK) | •<br>•<br>• | |

You should now have a small number of ticks beside items that you can really feel that it is worth acting on. Include strengths you want to make more use of as well as strengths you want to develop. These will be picked up in the action planning worksheets.

## 2.5    Preferences

This may be the most difficult area of all to get to grips with.  Why? Because few of us feel as if we can be put in a neat "box" to describe the sort of person we are.  We also are not necessarily consistent in our feelings and preferences.  In your more confident moments you may feel you are a reasonably outgoing individual.   In your bleaker moments you may feel anything but outgoing.

We are going to use a number of words to separate readily identifiable aspects of your personal characteristics.  The main headings will be:

- Social – what preferences we generally demonstrate in our relating to other people
- Thinking – the tendencies we demonstrate in solving problems, making decisions and creating plans
- Action – the preferences we demonstrate in the activities we pursue and the work we do
- Emotional – the underlying pattern of emotional reactions we experience

## Personality or Preferences?

Personality is usually defined in terms of the patterns of preferences we exhibit, although we might feel that some of our characteristics are based on aspects of ourselves that we have not chosen, in fact would rather not choose, and therefore shouldn't be thought of as a "preference", but rather as a "tendency".   According to Wikipedia:  "In psychology, personality is a collection of emotion, thought and behaviour patterns unique to a person."

For the purposes of your contentment project, it is more constructive and positive to think of our "Preferences", than to use the labels "tendencies" or "characteristics". An unusual aspect of the layout is that you will be able to score yourself positively on two apparently opposite preferences. This is designed to allow more room for our contradictory human natures – we can be both shy and outgoing – not at the same time, but in different circumstances – so let's be realistic about our complexity.

It can be extremely useful to be able to think about the circumstances where for example you are socially noisy, and those where you are quiet. If you are able to recognise what it is that affects your behaviour and how comfortable you feel, you are in a better position to either avoid the situations you dislike, or to do something about coping with them. The work-sheet will give you the space to rate yourself on each factor, and will also ask you to reflect on the resulting picture and to make notes on any apparent contradictions.

*John was middle-aged manager who found himself redundant and suffering a severe lack of confidence. Counselling sessions identified that sometimes he was able to display a very positive self-image and to behave and speak confidently. Other times he sounded and behaved in the opposite way. He was easily able to identify that he was a very different person when he wore the uniform of the voluntary armed service he belonged to. He had learned his technical duties and was able to instruct and lead others confidently. He confessed to the counsellor "I am a different person without the uniform." Some clear thinking about the circumstances that led to his uniformed confidence allowed him to replicate those in the rest of his life, and he developed a positive confidence that helped in the rest of his relationships. He didn't need to do anything dramatic other than recognise what was happening in the different sets of circumstances, and in a humorous way remind himself of his other self.*

You can decide that a preference is exactly how you want it to be, and be content to understand more clearly what suits you as an individual. You may decide that a preference that has become an unconscious habit is actually not how you want to be, and you can then go about changing it. This does not imply a huge change in your nature, but some people have for example found it really useful to learn to be more relaxed about meeting new people. Others have learned how to engage people in conversation, and found to their delight that it didn't hurt a bit.

The main headings and the definition of each factor or construct are as follows:

**Social**: The constructs that you will be able to score yourself on are:

- Outgoing – how easy you find it to relate to others, how likely you are to initiate conversations with others.
- Shy – how much you prefer not to be the focus of others' attention, how likely you are to avoid social contact.
- Noisy – how likely you are to contribute to conversations and to take a lead.
- Quiet – how likely you are to be content with listening to others without contributing.
- Dominant – how much you like to be in control, and to be able to manage the discussion.
- Agreeable – how important it is to you to be on good terms with others, and likely to compromise rather than argue.

**Thinking** – the constructs are

- Analytical – Do you think things through in a precise structured way?
- Gut feel – Do you decide quickly on the basis of what feels right?
- Detail – Do you pay attention to detail?
- Big picture – do you prefer to deal with broad views of issues?
- Structured – is your approach to mental activities structured, planned and orderly?
- Messy – do you prefer to take things as they come?
- Imaginative – do you like taking leaps of imagination and seeing things differently?
- Deductive – do you rely on logic to come to conclusions?

**Action** – the constructs are

- Individual – do you like to do things on your own?
- Group – do you prefer to work along with others?
- Practical – do you like to work on practical, physical things where you can see results?
- Theoretical – do you like to work on ideas and concepts?
- Artistic – do you like to be creative?
- People oriented – do you like the things you do to be helpful to others?
- Organised – do you plan and organise your activities?

**Emotions**: the constructs are

- Self-confidence – do you feel confident about yourself and your abilities?

- Optimism – do you generally take a positive view and expect good outcomes?
- Fragility – are you easily upset when things don't go well?
- Sensitivity – are you sensitive to other people's feelings and moods.
- Stability – are you generally good at coping with ups and downs of life?

Rate yourself on each of the factors on the worksheet. They are divided into Very low; low; average; high; very high. The numbers 1 – 10 allow you to rate yourself within those broad headings so that you create a personal profile for yourself. Remember that this isn't being imposed on you by anyone else, it is your honest rating of yourself – including any apparent contradictions. When you have completed it, look back over the ratings and fill in the comments box to highlight the factors that are either contradictory, or perhaps change depending on the circumstances you find yourself in.

**Social:**

| | V Low | | Low | | Average | | High | | V High | |
|---|---|---|---|---|---|---|---|---|---|---|
| | 1 | 2 | 3 | 4 | 5 | 6 | 7 | 8 | 9 | 10 |
| Outgoing | | | | | | | | | | |
| Shy | | | | | | | | | | |
| Noisy | | | | | | | | | | |
| Quiet | | | | | | | | | | |
| Dominant | | | | | | | | | | |
| Agreeable | | | | | | | | | | |

**Thinking**

| | V Low | | Low | | Average | | High | | V High | |
|---|---|---|---|---|---|---|---|---|---|---|
| | 1 | 2 | 3 | 4 | 5 | 6 | 7 | 8 | 9 | 10 |
| Analytical | | | | | | | | | | |
| Gut feel | | | | | | | | | | |
| Detail | | | | | | | | | | |
| Big picture | | | | | | | | | | |
| Structured | | | | | | | | | | |
| Messy | | | | | | | | | | |
| Imaginative | | | | | | | | | | |
| Deductive | | | | | | | | | | |

**Action**

| | V Low | | Low | | Average | | High | | V High | |
|---|---|---|---|---|---|---|---|---|---|---|
| | 1 | 2 | 3 | 4 | 5 | 6 | 7 | 8 | 9 | 10 |
| Individual | | | | | | | | | | |
| Group | | | | | | | | | | |
| Practical | | | | | | | | | | |
| Theoretical | | | | | | | | | | |
| Artistic | | | | | | | | | | |
| People oriented | | | | | | | | | | |
| Organised | | | | | | | | | | |

**Emotional**

| | V Low | | Low | | Average | | High | | V High | |
|---|---|---|---|---|---|---|---|---|---|---|
| | 1 | 2 | 3 | 4 | 5 | 6 | 7 | 8 | 9 | 10 |
| Self-confidence | | | | | | | | | | |
| Optimism | | | | | | | | | | |
| Fragility | | | | | | | | | | |
| Sensitivity | | | | | | | | | | |
| Stability | | | | | | | | | | |
| | | | | | | | | | | |

Notes

| Factor | Comment: (e.g. explaining circumstances, or apparent contradiction) |
|---|---|
| | |
| | |
| | |
| | |
| | |

## Psychometrics:

The scales that you have just used may remind you of the factors in some well-established psychometric instruments. If you want to pursue this way of gaining insight into yourself, and getting hold of good quality data about how you compare to other people, you will need to use a qualified practitioner. The scales in this book are deliberately simple and easy to apply to yourself in a common-sense way. If you want data that takes your insight further, make sure you use a qualified person who can help you interpret the complex data and avoid taking the wrong message from it.

## 2.6    Your dark side.


People are not always the individuals they want to be.  They sometimes lose their tempers.  Sometimes they are irrational.  Sometimes they may be stubborn beyond reason.  Sometimes they are upset and react strongly to something that on another day they would take in their stride.  These occasions which most of us would prefer not to happen are what we are calling your "dark side".

One of the most useful things we can do in relation to this less welcome part of our make-up is to understand it.  If we can look back on an outburst that we regret and analyse why it happened, we are well on the way to being able to either forgive ourselves for it or reduce the likelihood of it happening again.  Sometimes apparently negative reactions are actually helpful – either in revealing to ourselves how deeply we feel about something, or in registering with someone else just how strongly we feel about something.  The dark side isn't all bad.


**Using your history:**

When you filled in your "history line" earlier in this chapter, you will have identified highs and lows in your feelings during your adult life.  Use the worksheet below to analyse a number of the low points – picking particularly those when you reacted in a way that you would see as part of your dark side.  Some of the lows will probably be unavoidable, and your reactions may have been absolutely what you would expect.  The ones to pick for this exercise are those that with the benefit of hindsight you would now handle differently.  Try to pick only a few of them, and remember as you are doing it that this is a useful and positive exercise. Don't punish yourself all over again for what went wrong. Don't let yourself descend into the negative feelings again. Stand back and take an analytical look at what was happening to you – visualise it as a photograph or movie to distance yourself enough from it by looking through the camera.

| Incident | What in particular affected me? – Why? | Who was involved – what is significant about them? | What can I learn from it? |
|----------|----------------------------------------|----------------------------------------------------|---------------------------|
|          |                                        |                                                    |                           |
|          |                                        |                                                    |                           |
|          |                                        |                                                    |                           |

| Example | Example | Example | Example |
|---|---|---|---|
| **Incident** | **What in particular affected me? – Why?** | **Who was involved – what is significant about them?** | **What can I learn from it?** |
| *When I was depressed about the children, and we fought about school results and reports. They opted out of the family holiday.* | *I was furious that they weren't doing as well as I thought they could. Did I see a repeat of my own past?* | *The children; their mother; the friends we holiday with.*<br><br>*I saw myself isolated, with the children and their mother siding against me. It was enormously important to me that they did well.* | *My high expectations got in the way of me showing support and love. I created a barrier that was counterproductive. I need to be clear about my own need for them to excel, not impose it on them, and demonstrate more unconditional love to them.* |

Once again, you may find it easiest to work through this if you create a worksheet of your own on your computer or on a separate piece of paper.

That historical exercise will have allowed you to think about a few really significant "Downs". There are less significant ones day by day, but they are worth thinking about also. The next exercise involves thinking about a much shorter time-scale, and probably about less dramatic examples of the dark side. You are going to think back over the last few weeks – no more than 4, possibly fewer. This is an opportunity to think of the times when you were aware of a feeling, a reaction, or a behaviour that wasn't what you would choose.

| What happened? | What was **really** going on? | What can I learn from that? |
|---|---|---|
| **EXAMPLE** <br><br> *I became an indecisive mess over the present to buy for my mother-in-law, and argued unnecessarily.* | *In retrospect I was probably a bit resentful about the amount of money being spent, and I thought my partner's spontaneous generosity was wrong.* | *My careful and analytical nature gets in the way sometimes of my partner's enthusiasm! It also gets in the way of me making quick decisions. Perhaps I need to moderate it sometimes?* |
| **YOUR EXAMPLES** | | |
| | | |
| | | |

## The flip side of my strengths.

You will have identified strengths in the earlier section. We used the headings of Mental, Physical, Emotional, People, and Organisational. In your summary you will have picked some key strengths that are particularly important to you – not necessarily from all of the categories. Unfortunately every strength has a potential flip side. One person's self confidence can appear self-satisfied and smug to someone feeling vulnerable. Another person's strength in communicating effectively to a group can seem like dominance to the less confident. It is worth thinking about the potential for excess in each of our main strengths, and to think of the potential for negative impact on others – even though it is unintended.

**Examples**

| Strength | Flip side | Well? |
|---|---|---|
| *My ability to carefully analyse every detail.* | *Do I lose sight if the big picture? Do I annoy people who have grasped the general issue and want to move on?* | *Perhaps I should build in a pause to my detailed analysis when working with others. Check if they want me to do it separately and move on?* |
| *My ability to think ahead and plan activities in detail.* | *Do I miss opportunities for just saying "yes" and trying something new? Do I drive people mad who like to be spontaneous?* | *Yes I do! While not wanting to let go of this strength I could at least assess if I'm always using it well. There are times it doesn't matter.* |

| Strength | Flip-side | Well? |
|---|---|---|
|  |  |  |
|  |  |  |
|  |  |  |
|  |  |  |

## 2.7    Ongoing self-review.

As you will have found in working your way through this chapter, it is not easy or quick to really think about yourself and analyse what is going on. It can even be a tiring and stressful activity. Perhaps that is why most people are not very good at doing it.

Now that you have extracted a structured set of reflections about yourself, you have the basis for keeping it under review.

### Using the data:

The reflections and summaries you have created in this chapter are going to be really useful in the rest of your Contentment Project. As you work your way through each of the chapters you will find you need to refer back to the lists of strengths and to remind yourself of what you have been able to say about the complex, possibly contradictory mixture of abilities and emotions that make up your nature. You have to know yourself well before you can make realistic plans and good decisions.

### Solo vs Shared:

This book is designed to give enough prompting headings and enough examples for you to complete it on your own. However, many people find that sharing their thoughts and conclusions helps to put them in perspective. It is also very useful to have a trusted person's reaction to your statements. It really is helpful for you to gather comments from other people if you are going to be totally confident about your picture. A comment from a trusted friend that "yes, we all do rely on you to be the careful thinker about anything financial," will serve to confirm and strengthen the picture you have been able to build up yourself.

An ideal situation would be for a small group – probably only 3 people – who have all used the book, to organise a review together from time to time. It is extremely positive, if you have been trying to develop some of your behaviours, for you to receive feedback that someone has noticed. It is also a worthwhile discipline to have an occasion when you have to explain to others your analysis of your strengths and development.

So chose for yourself- as both methods are valid. Just make sure you do it!


## Frequency:

The ideal frequency depends on you. Most people find that it is unhelpful to undertake as serious a review as this more frequently than once per year. You may like to have some progress-checks with others if you are able to work as a pair or group, but a really thorough review probably should not be too frequent. Some people find that the New Year holiday provides both the time and the inclination to engage in a personal review. Others find that an existing pattern – for example the autumn walking holiday – provides a good opportunity with an established timing for doing the thinking.

Whatever the choice you make, try to plan it ahead. Try to resolve when it will be useful to you to revisit it. Depending on your preferences some of you will right away put a note in your diary. Others will prefer to wait until the mood is right. Whatever your style, use the headings and keep reflecting and learning.

# Chapter 3 Values

## Sections in Chapter 3

**3.1 Values**

**3.2 Gathering the evidence**

**3.3 How you use your time**

**3.4 Making decisions**

**3.5 Losing sleep**

**3.6 Recognising influences**

**3.7 Family**

**3.8 Influential others**

**3.9 Heroes and Villains**

**3.10 Religious belief**

**3.11 Integrating your review**

**3.12 Worksheets**

- Time analysis
- Decision analysis
- Worry analysis
- Family influence
- Other influence
- Heroes and villains

# Chapter 3

## 3.1   Values

Consciously or not, we all operate to a set of values. Even if you have never used the word, or devoted a second to thinking about them, you have a set of values that are of enormous significance in how you run your life.

Values are the "things that are important to us." They influence us every minute of every day. They affect the little everyday decisions we make just as they influence the more obviously momentous decisions. Even if we are completely unaware of them, they are at work in our every move. Like habits they become more and more ingrained and exert more and more power over us. So they are worth paying attention to. Strangely enough, like the noise we are exposed to every day, we may no longer be conscious of them, but that makes them stronger rather than weaker, as they influence our lives unchallenged if we do not stop to think what they really are.

One of the deceptive things about Values is that they don't have to be articulated to have their power. Putting them into words is part of the process of getting to grips with them. Leaving them unspoken is a certain way to leave us at their mercy. It is only through devoting some time to identifying what our values really are that we can consciously manage them and manage the way we are living our lives.

Values sound noble and worthwhile, but they can equally be selfish, ignoble, and destructive. The rules that operate in a criminal gang are a set of values for the members. They determine how people react to each other, and form the basis of deciding what behaviour is acceptable and what is not. The code that exists in the criminal gang may be very different to the one that you aspire to, and if so you will more easily recognise it as an expression of priorities very different from your own. It is easier to recognise sets of values different from our own than it is to be conscious of what we take for granted every day. That doesn't mean that what we take for granted is what we would choose if we really thought about it. Nor does it mean that it is the best that we could choose. However it is what we have chosen by default as the set of things that are important to us, and unconsciously we allow them to build into a framework that influences all that we do.

This chapter will help you to analyse the evidence that exposes the Values you are using. It will also lead you through some systematic thinking about the Values you would like to have. It will try to make conscious the things that have not been articulated, and give you the opportunity to decide what is right for you.

## 3.2    Gathering the evidence:

The introductory statements to this chapter suggest that all of us every day are doing things on the basis of the internal, invisible, and generally unconscious code of Values that we have adopted. There are many potential ways of tackling the business of making clear, visible and conscious the rules that are driving us. Stop the average person in the street and ask them "What are your Values?" and you are unlikely to be able to extract a coherent or accurate picture. Similarly if you were to try to write a list of your six key values they could be more of a wish-list than a reflection of reality. You may be one of the few who genuinely are behaving and living the way you would aspire to.  For most of us we need to be helped to look at the reality.  The most revealing starting point is to look at the hard evidence.

*Valerie is a very dynamic manager.  She runs a unit in the public sector health service, and has seen it through difficult times with great success.  She is married, early forties, and lives in comfortable style in south London.  Asked about her values she volunteered a list that included Honesty; Lack of Prejudice; Environmental Awareness; Family Values; and Generosity.  Embarrassed at the extent to which they sounded like a political manifesto, she agreed to some exploration of the evidence.*

*We discussed the previous working week and the weekend that followed it, looking at the way that she spent her time, the decisions she had made, and the highs and lows of the week.*

*Time had been spent at work doing things other than what she wanted.  She confessed that she had spent a lot of time on technical issues when she had discovered that things were not going according to plan in a major planning project.  Once warmed up in describing the week, she became animated and passionate not only about the technical issue, but also about the failings of her colleagues who had allowed things to go wrong.  She had worked long hours putting things right, had taken the project from her colleague and kept her boss happy.  The more we talked about the horrors of the week, the more she confessed about the blazing rows with her colleague, the excuses that she had to invent for her boss, and the frequency with which this pattern emerged.  The analysis continued for some time, and we wrote on a flip-chart some of the key words and themes that were emerging.*

*I then asked Valerie to look at the flip-chart as though it had been written about another person — someone she had not met — and to speculate about the set of Values that drove that imaginary individual. To her dismay Valerie found herself listing a set of words that were very different from the original set of aspirational values. Words included Competitive; Perfectionist; Putting her work first; and finally Selfish.*

*In a painful session, Valerie came to realise that unwittingly she had become someone she never meant to be. Driven by a need to succeed and to prove herself, she had allowed the needs of the job to over-ride all the other Values that she had thought she had. For what seemed like good reasons and for "the good of the unit" she had become less than honest, she was difficult to work for, and she routinely insulted and harangued her colleagues. Putting into words the conclusions from a look at the evidence gave Valerie a devastating insight into the person she had become. It was painful for her, but it gave her the basis for a serious re-think about the way she handled her work, the way she dealt with her colleagues, and the way she used her time.*

Hopefully you will not have as traumatic a revelation as Valerie about the Values that actually drive you. But whatever they are, your only way of reasserting control over who you are is to use some honest analysis and reflection to find out what has been happening.

## 3.3  How you use your time

The example of Valerie gives a clue about the power of looking at the hard facts.  This exercise will help you to carry out a simple analysis and to draw some conclusions from what you find.

It is important to look not at what "in principle" you think happens, but at what really did happen over a period of time.  The exercise asks you to look at the last week, but you can modify this if necessary.

The following example of 2 days' analysis should give an idea of the sort of detail, and the sort of conclusions that may be possible.  Once again – this is not the sort of analysis that you would do for publication to your boss or to your colleagues.  It needs to be honest and based on what you really did.

The example is of a working person called Jack – in this case someone who works in an office, and with a high degree of freedom to decide hour by hour what he does.  However the same principles apply if you are not in paid employment, if you are in a very restrictive job, or if you are self-employed.  The answers will look different from the example, but the principle is the same.

|  |  | Significant activity | What does that tell me? |
|---|---|---|---|
| Monday | 0700 - 0900 | Breakfast and driving | Routine - not ecologically sound! |
| | 0900 - 1300 | Phone calls, mail, 2 meetings | Sounds not very dynamic! Reactive? |
| | 1300 - 1700 | Lunch with Liz, internet search for holiday flights, phone with Dave, arranging car service. | Use of time? Am I using work time well? |
| | 1700 - 2100 | Driving, reading paper, eating, tv | Sounds boring, and not energetic or helpful |
| | 2100 - 2400 | tv, bed | same again |
| | 2400 - 0700 | ? | ? |
| Tuesday | 0700 - 0900 | Breakfast and driving | Definitely routine |
| | 0900 - 1300 | Phone calls, mail, agenda for Wed meeting, time with Barney, sorting printer | Doing what has to be done. Reactive then taking refuge in what I like doing (tech issues)? |
| | 1300 - 1700 | Working on printer, phone calls about Wed | Not what I'm paid for! |
| | 1700 - 2100 | Driving, reading paper, eating, tv | As above |
| | 2100 - 2400 | tv, bed | As above |
| | 2400 - 0700 | ? | |

So what conclusions does Jack (our imaginary reviewer) draw about himself?

| | What is important to this person? | |
|---|---|---|
| 1 | | *I am being reactive about work, doing what I have to and taking refuge in things that I enjoy.* |
| 2 | | *My own personal needs and interests are given room in work* |
| 3 | | *Contributing at home doesn't seem to be a routine value that drives my behaviour.* |
| 4 | | |
| 5 | | |
| 6 | | |

So far these are probably a little harsh, but if he keeps up the analysis for a couple of weeks a more definite picture will emerge. This analysis is only one of the series to uncover your operating Values. The next one is about significant decisions that you have made recently, and the final one is about things that have really bothered you – perhaps kept you awake at night.

Take time now to complete the time analysis sheets on page 75 & 76 before moving on to the next section. Try also to fill in the section which asks you to draw conclusions about the pattern of use of time.

**Pretend it is someone else!**

Look at the record of the use of time as if it is not you. Only by being really dispassionate about it are you able to draw useful conclusions. Without taking into account that you know you are really a deeply caring and considerate individual, and that on various occasions you have sweated blood for your business, what does the cold look at last week's use of time tell you?

## 3.4   Making Decisions

This section is going to ask you to think back over the last few months and list a number of decisions that were important to you. Depending on the sorts of things you do, important can mean infinitely different things. Each of us has our own range of issues that we have freedom to make decisions about, and sometimes we don't value our own decision-making scope. However big or small the decisions may seem, they are just as useful as raw material for thinking about what is important to you.

Don't worry about making firm conclusions at this stage. Looking back over the few decisions the form allows you will prompt you to ask yourself questions - for example "does this mean I put work before all else...?" or "does this mean I am willing to be economical with the truth now?". You will be able to decide when you have completed all three exercises.

The following example shows just two decisions and the reflections that followed.

| | What was the decision? | What factors did I pay attention to? | What does this tell me about my values? |
|---|---|---|---|
| Decision 1 | I decided that we would go for a four-week holiday in the summer. | I thought about how much we had enjoyed longer holidays in the past, and weighed up the cost against what we would save in living expenses here. | I didn't take into account my elderly mother and the extra demand on my sister looking after her. It seems to show I put more emphasis on my wishes than on the effect on others? |
| | **What was the decision?** | **What factors did I pay attention to?** | **What does this tell me about my values?** |
| Decision 2 | I decided that I wouldn't argue with my colleague over the office business plan, even though I didn't believe it would work. | I paid attention to my aversion to another row, and to the amount of extra work and argument that would follow if I objected. | Have I become more interested in the quiet life than in maintaining standards? Am I allowing things to happen that ideally I should be objecting to? |
| | **What was the decision?** | **What factors did I pay attention to?** | **What does this tell me about my values?** |
| Decision 3 | | | |

When Jack comes to answer the questions at the bottom of the page he feels pretty negative about this individual he is looking at:

| | What is important to this person? | | |
|---|---|---|---|
| 1 | He puts himself first. His pleasure has become more important than his family. | | |
| 2 | He values the quiet life - doesn't seem to be driven by other principles. | | |
| 3 | | | |
| 4 | | | |

The other exercises may allow him to balance the negative evidence here with some more positive features later.

Fill in the decision worksheet on page 77 at the end of the chapter now. Try to fill in 3 or 4 decisions, and then try to answer dispassionately, "What is important to this person?"

## 3.5   Losing sleep (or those worrying worries)

Perhaps you do not lose sleep over any worries.  If so, you are one of a very fortunate minority.  Most people experience worries that interfere with sleep. Occasional sleeplessness is perfectly normal and not to be worried about. Only very frequent disturbances are a cause for concern.

The things that waken us at 5:00 in the morning can be very useful indicators of issues that need to be addressed, and can also give a useful insight into our Values.  Interestingly they may need a little interpretation to see beyond the immediate cause. The following example illustrates the point.

*John is a 50-ish professional.  He works long hours, and needs to be out of bed by 0645 each day and ready for work by 0800.  He found that he was experiencing annoying sleep disturbances, and noticed that they occurred both early in the night and the hours before time to get up.  As a result, he was not feeling well rested, and was increasingly conscious that he was not performing at his best.  The cumulative pattern was having a serious affect on his attitude to work, and on his belief in himself as a competent performer.  When questioned about what was going through his mind when he found himself tossing and turning he reported a variety of work tasks.  They were largely troublesome details that he needed to remember to take care of, or niggles about the preparation for formal sessions that he was about to present.  The usual remedies of sitting up to make a note of the specific issues so that he could relax as they were on the list for the morning didn't seem to work.  Each time he dealt with one set of niggles, others arose to take their place.*

*Longer conversation revealed that the detail was almost irrelevant; he could never get to the end of the list. There was an underlying theme however, which was about his belief in the value of the work. He had found himself with an area of work which was not his choosing, and he did not really feel at ease. He was theoretically well qualified for it, but it did not seem worthwhile to him, - it didn't appeal to his sense of contributing to society. What seemed to be disturbing him was not so much the host of details that he needed to remember, but rather the suppressed worry that his career was going off-track because he was doing work that he didn't believe in.*

*Fortunately he was able to discuss the issue with his colleagues and arrange to go back to his original area of work, which gave him a much greater feeling of satisfaction. The little voices wakening him in the night had not been caused by the annoying details he had to remember to fix. They had been caused by a much more fundamental worry that he wasn't living up to some deeply held Values about working in an area that made a social contribution. The niggles that troubled him were not earth-shattering in themselves, but because they were not fitting in with his unexpressed but deeply held Values, they were disproportionately annoying. The fact that they were so unreasonably disturbing was the clue to think about what was really behind the disturbance.*

This example hopefully gives a clue about how you may need to dig beneath the surface of the worry that keeps you awake. For the purposes of this chapter, what we are looking for is the Value that you hold which is making the specific issue so significant. If you identify that you were disturbed because you had not been able to find the right present for your child's birthday – the conclusion should not be that you are a particularly fussy shopper, or that your local shops are not good enough, but rather that "doing the very best you can for your children" is a strong Value that you need to find ways to express.    If you were annoyed by the scratch on your child's new bicycle, what analysis do you make of your reaction?  The issue may not be the specific of the condition of the paintwork on the bicycle, nor of the effect on the resale value of the bicycle.  However it may well give you pause to reflect on that highly developed Value you place on keeping things in perfect condition.

If you bring that out and look at it as a Value, you may well come to conclude that something you have allowed to carry over from your own childhood has become an inappropriate and anachronistic Value that causes you quite unreasonable anguish.  The fact that you have never put this into words doesn't mean that it isn't having an influence on your thoughts and on your reactions.  You may be more critical of your children than you ideally would like to be.  You may be more fussy about the condition of your car than you think in your relaxed moments you really should be.  But you are driven by that Value whether you like it or not.

This chapter and the worksheet that follows give you the opportunity to identify the Values that lie behind your reactions, and to think about their relevance to you now.  There is space to think about four worries that have bothered you.  You may find all the evidence you need from two or three of them.

## Sample Worry Worksheet

| | What was the worry? | What was going on in my head? | What is the underlying Value this reveals? |
|---|---|---|---|
| Worry 1 | I was worried that the toy pram we bought for Joanna's birthday wasn't a good enough present. | I worry about doing the best I can for my children. I suppose it wasn't really the detail of the toy pram, but more a feeling of dissatisfaction with my parenting. | The value must be connected to "doing the very best I can for my children". |
| | What was the worry? | What was going on in my head? | What is the underlying Value this reveals? |
| Worry 2 | I was enormously annoyed by the scratch on the side of the car as a result of Jane's driving | I hate to see anything damaged. I spend a lot of time cleaning and polishing the car and am the same about all my possessions. At the time that seemed more important than Jane's hurt feelings or the effect on our relationship. | "Keeping possessions as good as new" sounds pathetic but seems to come through when I think of what bothers me. |

## Sample Reflection on the Worry Worksheet:

| | What is important to this person? |
|---|---|
| 1 | Doing the very best for my children |
| 2 | Keeping all my possessions in perfect "as new" condition |
| 3 | |
| 4 | |

This raw material gives you the chance to think about the extent to which the Values that emerge from the analysis are really the Values that you want to have in your life.

Fill in the Worry Worksheet on page 78 now. Take time to think about what is really behind the worries, then again answer "What is really important to this person?"

## 3.6    Recognising the influences on our Values

We all are subject to influences, some of us more easily influenced than others. This applies to our Values just as much as to any other aspect of life. Have you thought systematically about who has influenced you and in what way? This section will give you a simple way of thinking about the people who have influenced you; to think about the nature of that influence, and to check the importance of it. You will be trying to put into words influences that are real and are affecting you every day. Thinking about them and analysing them gives you the opportunity to be aware of what is happening and gives you the opportunity to exercise some control over them. If you don't do this, they will carry on anyway – you just won't be aware of it!

The worksheets will give you the opportunity to think in an organised way about some different categories of people that have influenced you. We will use just three general categories – your immediate family, the adults you have interacted with, and the more distant historical, fictional, or mythical figures that populate your mind.

Influences work in both positive and negative ways. You will be thinking of the ways in which you have reacted against someone's influence just as much as you will be thinking about how you try to live up to a hero's example. Rather like our reaction to the Values of the criminal gang, it is often easier to recognise what we do not want to be like than to identify the positive example.

## 3.7 Family:

The first worksheet asks you to think about family influences. Don't worry if your family isn't the conventional shape and size. Whoever you spent time with as you were growing up, who had responsibility for you, and who you looked to for your security and "foundation". In the following example the influences are the very conventional Father, Mother, and Grandfather. Use the sheet to insert those who are genuinely relevant to you.

**Sample family influence sheet:**

| Family | | | | |
|---|---|---|---|---|
| Who | Key features that influenced me | How did that to affect me? | Is this OK? | Action? |
| My father | Probably his energy - always active and getting on with things. | This probably is one of the reasons why I feel guilty if I'm lazy! I disapprove of my own or others' idleness. | Yes - this is OK for me, but I maybe disapprove too much. | * |
| My mother | Her excessive politeness and unwillingness to inconvenience people. | Made me impatient and I react against dithering! | No - I have gone too far the other way. | * |
| Grandfather | His modesty and understatement. I gradually discovered the positively exciting life he had led. | Impressed me mightily. Made me dissatisfied with unexciting life. | Yes - good stimulus - but not doing enough about it! | * |

All three of the family influences here have an asterisk in the "Action" column. Jack (our sample worksheet user) recognises the extent to which his father's energy set an example for him which has led to a Value about "Always being active – never being idle", which while praiseworthy in many ways can lead to guilty feelings and to disapproving of others who have a more laid-back style. He recognises that he needs to think about this and build it in to the later integration exercise

He recognises also that his mother's excessive politeness used to annoy him. He can remember thinking she could never give a straight answer even if asked if she would like a cup of tea! He remembers how he used to react against it and as a result became too outspokenly firm and impolite. He needs to reflect on the extent to which that old habit still affects the way he responds to others. He has a suspicion that a Value to do with "speak your mind even if it upsets people" is no longer useful or desirable.

Finally he remembers the extent to which he was impressed to learn as a teenager about the exciting life that his grandfather had led. Wars and travel had been a major part of his grandfather's young life – and left an example that was hard to follow. The Value that seemed to be lurking in his mind was about the "importance of being a risk-taker", and the dissatisfaction with a life that seemed too conventional and safe. His reflections on this lead him to realise that there is some unfinished business in his mind. If this is a value he really does want to hold, then he either needs to get on with doing something a little less conventional and a bit more daring, or he will live with a vague sense of dissatisfaction with himself. Alternatively, having a serious look at the Value might lead him to conclude that his world wasn't really like that anymore, and that the unfavourable comparison of himself with his grandfather was an unhelpful burden. He could rejoice in the exploits of the old man without feeling that it was necessary to emulate them!

Complete the Family worksheet on page 79 before progressing to the next section.

## 3.8   Influential Others:

The worksheet asks you to identify a small number of the people you have come across, and perhaps still relate to, who made an impression on you. Once again the reaction can be a positive one that leads you to want to emulate the individual, or it may have been a negative reaction that makes it less likely that you will feel comfortable following that example.

| Other | | | | |
|-------|--------------------------------|--------------------|------------|----------|
| Who | Key features that influenced me | How did that affect me? | Is this OK? | Action? |
| KG | He was a totally principled man, who was a great headmaster but also a delightful human being. | A bit awe-inspiring, but the combination of humanity and principle is a good model to follow. | Yes I'd love to follow this example | Lot of work to do!  * |

Thinking about, and whittling down to a small number of the people that have made the greatest impact is a difficult-sounding task.   Don't worry at this stage!   If you can identify around 3 – 6 people and their influence for good or bad, that will give sufficient input for now.   There will be opportunities in the future to re-visit the exercise and test out the addition of other people.

Our example "KG", leads Jack to think about the extent to which he is able to live up to the example he has identified.  In the integration stage at the end of the book, he will be able to build this in to the action planning – and you will find some practical hints about how to consciously make use of the positive examples you decide you would like to emulate.

Complete the "Other" worksheet on page 80 now before going on to the last section.

## 3.9    Heroes and villains

Time to let the imagination run a little more freely.  This worksheet gives the opportunity to identify the people you haven't met, who are historical figures or even who exist only in fiction, but whose influence you know has had an effect on you.  Once again they can be negative examples – people whose Values you would want to ensure that you could never be suspected of holding.

Jack in this example thinks of two well known European public figures who had opposite effects on him.  He probably argued about them with friends, but hadn't thought in an organised way about the implications of his views.

**Hero/myth/fiction**

| Who | Key features that influenced me | How did that affect me? | Is this OK? | Action? |
|---|---|---|---|---|
| Margaret Thatcher | Her belief that "society" didn't exist, just a collection of self-interested individuals. | Repulsion!  Made me determined to hang on to a belief that people are better than that, and unselfishness does exist! | Still very important, but I'm not doing anything about it. | * |
| Mary Robinson | Her unselfish energy to "do things"!  When she could have been quietly wealthy and comfortable she persisted with public service. | Admiration.  The antidote to MT. Made me want to have some form of altruistic activity in my life. | Still an important aspiration - but no action. | * |

Jack reacted very differently to the two people – but the message from both is consistent.  The asterisks in the Action column mean that Jack is going to need to carry this evidence forward when he is reviewing his set of Values.

Complete the Heroes and Villains worksheet on page 81 now.  Take your time to reflect on it and think about the historic, fictional or mythical figures that have influenced you.  Ask yourself if the influence is OK, and mark the Action column if you think you need to do more about that influence.  You will be able to build the action points into the final exercise in the chapter.

## 3.10  Religious belief

For some of you the absence of reference to religious belief as a basis for Values may have been puzzling.  You may have the view that your religion provides you with the set of Values that you need. What this exercise will do is to give the opportunity to integrate the code of Values that you may adopt through your religion with the Values that you arrive at as an individual human being.

There is no conflict between having strongly held religious belief and thinking out Values for yourself.  You may find the religious input a good starting point, and find the exercises give greater depth and practicality in application of the Values.  Rather than undermining any strongly held beliefs, the exercises in this chapter should help to strengthen, confirm and refresh what is important to you.

Fortunately it also works for those with other "codes" that influence their Values.  A Humanist can use the chapter just as successfully and usefully as a Monk, an Agnostic or an Atheist.

The positive usefulness for anyone in tackling the analysis of their Values, is that an organised review gives the opportunity to look at them, check their relevance, and check the extent to which they are being reflected in our daily lives.  A common reaction is to find a strengthening of the Values that we aspire to, and a pleasure in the process of putting them into words. The "Action" column gives a clear prompt about the need to demonstrate Values in practice.  Values that can not be observed in your behaviour are not really Values at all.   The link between the final section of this chapter (Integrating the worksheets into a coherent statement of Values) and the following chapter (identifying Purpose, Objectives and Plans) is crucial.  Your contentment project is a holistic review of your life, but the emphasis is firmly on turning aspirations into practical realities.

## 3.11  Integrating your review of your Values

This chapter has contained a large number of worksheets.  Do not be surprised if some of them have appealed to you more than others.  Some may have been easy, natural and pleasurable to complete.  Others will probably have seemed like hard work to you.  The next stage is the exciting one, where you extract from all the data you have created a short list of the key factors.   You will then create your Value statement, which is simply saying  *"I want to organise my life and make my decisions on the basis of ......"*

STEP 1

You should have three summary sheets looking like this from the Time, Decision, and Worry worksheets.

| | What is important to this person? |
|---|---|
| 1 | |
| 2 | |
| 3 | |
| 4 | |
| 5 | |
| 6 | |

You will probably have filled in most of the lines in each of the three. Hopefully they have given you the basis for an interesting review of your use of time, your decisions, and your worries, and what that tells you about yourself. The "standing outside yourself and looking at the data as if at a stranger" is particularly relevant here.

Having read the three lists now combine them into the "What is Really Important?" table. This will require a bit of thought and reflection. Take your time so that you have a list that is based on evidence and that the imaginary stranger observing you could confirm. Do this now.

| | What is *really* important to this person? |
|---|---|
| 1 | |
| 2 | |
| 3 | |
| 4 | |
| 5 | |
| 6 | |

STEP 2

You will also have your 3 Worksheets from the "Influence" section. One dealing with Family influence, one with Other People, and one with your Heroes & Villains. Look at the **"Is this OK" and "Action"** columns to pick up on the influences that you want to build in to your statement.

Take time to think about each of those influences and then complete the following table. It allows you to list the things that you would like to see as part of this person that is the YOU we are examining. You may have found in the analysis of your time, decisions and worries that you have an operational set of Values that are not exactly as you would like them. The reflection on the Influences will have given you the opportunity to think about the positive influences and examples that you would like to have a features in your Values in the future. It will also have given you the opportunity to identify the negative examples that you want to make sure that you do not emulate.

Having reflected on those influences, now fill in the following table with the features you would like to ensure that you have in your Values in future. (Again the question is phrased impersonally so that you can look at yourself as if you are a dispassionate observer – rather than as yourself!)

| | What I **want** to be important to this person? |
|---|---|
| 1 | |
| 2 | |
| 3 | |
| 4 | |
| 5 | |
| 6 | |

STEP 3

You now have two short lists of things that (a) you have demonstrated are Values driving your behaviour, and (b) are Values demonstrated by people who have influenced you, that you would like to build in to your personal Values.

The really crucial step now is to combine those into your statement of Values. This can be aspirational – in other words you can get beyond what you have been demonstrating in your life so far, and start to build the way you want to be.

A good way of starting each Value statement is "I want to run my life on the basis of......."

Try the table below as a means of integrating the thinking you have completed in this chapter. You will find Jack's example of his first few new Value statements first.

| | I want to run my life on the basis of: |
|---|---|
| 1 | Giving time and attention to my family and avoiding work taking over time that is for them. |
| 2 | Contributing socially outside the family, to the wider community |
| 3 | Living up to my standard of honesty and integrity in all I do |
| 4 | Being a good friend and colleague, who listens and helps. |
| 5 | Being innovative and adventurous; finding new things to do and getting out of the rut |
| 6 | Valuing people over possessions. |

And now the blank table for you to fill in. Try to make it reflect the most important items you have identified in your summary tables – but remember – this is how you want things to be from now on!

| | I want to run my life on the basis of: |
|---|---|
| 1 | |
| 2 | |
| 3 | |
| 4 | |
| 5 | |
| 6 | |

## 3.12  Worksheets:

1. Time analysis

2. Decision analysis

3. Worry analysis

4. Family influence worksheet

5. Other influence worksheet

6. Heroes and villains worksheet

# Time analysis:

| | | Significant activity | What does that tell me? |
|---|---|---|---|
| Monday | 0700 - 0900 | | |
| | 0900 - 1300 | | |
| | 1300 - 1700 | | |
| | 1700 - 2100 | | |
| | 2100 - 2400 | | |
| | 2400 - 0700 | | |
| Tuesday | 0700 - 0900 | | |
| | 0900 - 1300 | | |
| | 1300 - 1700 | | |
| | 1700 - 2100 | | |
| | 2100 - 2400 | | |
| | 2400 - 0700 | | |
| Wednesday | 0700 - 0900 | | |
| | 0900 - 1300 | | |
| | 1300 - 1700 | | |
| | 1700 - 2100 | | |
| | 2100 - 2400 | | |
| | 2400 - 0700 | | |
| Thursday | 0700 - 0900 | | |
| | 0900 - 1300 | | |
| | 1300 - 1700 | | |
| | 1700 - 2100 | | |
| | 2100 - 2400 | | |
| | 2400 - 0700 | | |

| | | | |
|---|---|---|---|
| Friday | 0700 - 0900 | | |
| | 0900 - 1300 | | |
| | 1300 - 1700 | | |
| | 1700 - 2100 | | |
| | 2100 - 2400 | | |
| | 2400 - 0700 | | |
| Saturday | 0700 - 0900 | | |
| | 0900 - 1300 | | |
| | 1300 - 1700 | | |
| | 1700 - 2100 | | |
| | 2100 - 2400 | | |
| | 2400 - 0700 | | |
| Sunday | 0700 - 0900 | | |
| | 0900 - 1300 | | |
| | 1300 - 1700 | | |
| | 1700 - 2100 | | |
| | 2100 - 2400 | | |
| | 2400 - 0700 | | |

| | What is important to this person? |
|---|---|
| 1 | |
| 2 | |
| 3 | |
| 4 | |
| 5 | |
| 6 | |

# Decision analysis worksheet:

| | What was the decision? | What factors did I pay attention to? | What does this tell me about my values? |
|---|---|---|---|
| Decision 1 | | | |
| Decision 2 | | | |
| Decision 3 | | | |
| Decision 4 | | | |
| Decision 5 | | | |

| | What is important to this person? |
|---|---|
| 1 | |
| 2 | |
| 3 | |
| 4 | |
| 5 | |
| 6 | |

## Worry worksheet:

| | What was the worry? | What was going on in my head? | What is the underlying Value this reveals? |
|---|---|---|---|
| Worry 1 | | | |
| Worry 2 | | | |
| Worry 3 | | | |
| Worry 4 | | | |

| | What is important to this person? |
|---|---|
| 1 | |
| 2 | |
| 3 | |
| 4 | |
| 5 | |
| 6 | |

# Family influence worksheet

| Family | | | | | |
|--------|--------|--------|--------|--------|--------|
| Who | Key features that influenced me | How did that affect me? | Is this OK? | Action? | |
|  |  |  |  |  | |
|  |  |  |  |  | |
|  |  |  |  |  | |
|  |  |  |  |  | |

## Other influence worksheet

| Other | Who | Key features that influenced me | How did that affect me? | Is this OK? | Action? |
|---|---|---|---|---|---|
| | | | | | |
| | | | | | |
| | | | | | |
| | | | | | |
| | | | | | |

**Heroes and Villains influence worksheet**

| Hero/Myth/Fiction | | | | |
|---|---|---|---|---|
| Who | Key features that influenced me | How did that affect me? | Is this OK? | Action? |
| | | | | |
| | | | | |
| | | | | |
| | | | | |
| | | | | |

# Notes

# Chapter 4

# Purpose and plans

## Sections in Chapter 4

# Chapter 4

## 4.1    Purpose and Plans

*What good am I if I know and don't do*
*If I see and don't say if I look right through you*
*If I turn a deaf ear to the thunderin' sky*
*What good am I?*

*Bob Dylan*

"Events, dear boy, events," was how Harold Macmillan succinctly expressed the major factor in thwarting his best intentions.  He was thoughtfully aware of how his most carefully crafted plans could be sabotaged, undermined, and rendered irrelevant by simple "things that happen".

Life seems to conspire to make sure that there are too many events hitting us day by day to allow us to conduct our lives in an orderly pre-planned way, or even in the relaxed laid-back style we might prefer. Whether it is an unexpected illness, a car that fails to start, or a sudden storm, events that we cannot control often rearrange our priorities and determine what we have to do today.

The "arrogance of planning" is brought home to us so frequently that some of us run the risk of giving up.  People refuse to plan too far ahead because they were disappointed in a previous plan.  A sharp reminder from fickle fate of our vulnerability can leave us disillusioned about the value of planning and setting objectives. I have even experienced people who quote religious reasons for avoiding any form of planning.

However the absence of planning is disabling. Avoiding setting objectives condemns us to the absence of feelings of achievement. Without any plans or targets we end up without a feeling of purpose. The gnawing feeling of purposelessness is one of the most depressing and disabling that afflicts us. "What's the point?", is one of the most frequent phrases from the depressed and disillusioned.

The previous chapter will have helped you to think about "what is important to me". The final exercise will have enabled you to create your statements based on the phrase "I want to live my life on the basis of...." Those statements are enormously important. They can evolve and be refined as we live and experience, and can be the foundation on which plans can be built. They provide the touch-stone that helps decision making and that gives perspective in confusion and perplexity. They are a crucial element in managing your way to Contentment, but they are not enough.

Dylan's words are a taunting challenge to us to put good intentions into action. What good are we if we are conscious of how we should live our lives but don't do so? What good are we if we take the time to think about and articulate the basis on which we want to run our lives, but don't actually take the action that is needed to turn it into reality?

This chapter is about clarifying what we want to do in our lives, and about planning in a way that is realistic and sufficiently robust to survive "Events".

## 4.2   Broad vs Precise

The title for this section could equally well be Themes vs Specifics. The key message is about the real practical possibility of planning in a way that is worthwhile and liveable.   The contrast can maybe be highlighted in two opposing examples:

*James is a list person.  He not only has lists of things to do today, he has lists of everything.  He is a convert to the life-planning process and has set himself a challenging list of "things to achieve" along with dates and deadlines.  He has decided to take up Judo, and plans to achieve his Green Belt by the end of the year.   In the interests of a balanced life he is also going to exercise his mind, and has joined a reading group which he plans to lead forward into a doubling of membership.*

*Poor James.  He finds that the reading group doesn't conform to his plan.   The current members are very happy with the size of the group, resent his pushy intervention, and pointedly ignore his offer to organise things.  Meanwhile the local Judo class is postponed when the instructor is injured, and James ends up feeling "what's the point in all this planning?"*

*Julie meanwhile has taken a different approach.   She completed her statements of "I want to live my life on the basis of....." and decided that she would identify something that allowed her to contribute to the community as a priority this year.  Meanwhile she would try to spot opportunities to turn the other themes she had identified into practical action.   One was about her physical well-being, and the other about developing her role as daughter to her elderly father.*

*Julie's initial action plan was broad and open to opportunities. She was disappointed at first with her lack of progress in identifying a community contribution. However a downturn in her father's health led her to put some real effort into developing a new and rewarding relationship with him. She started to learn what it meant to be a carer, and turned her old grudgingly dutiful daughter role into a positive and developmental one. She started a project with him to document the family history, and every week they tried to add some more details to the growing file. The old man's doctor noticed the change in the father's mood, and asked Julie to meet with some other carers to share thoughts and experience in looking after the elderly. Before long Julie's "Themes" were all being given an opportunity for practical expression. She had not been able to plan it all in detail, but by being clear about the themes or components she wanted, she was able to recognise them and grasp them when they appeared.*

Those examples are perhaps a little obvious, but the message is a serious one. It can be summarised in four key points:

1. Creating plans and objectives, on the basis of our Values, is a necessary step towards feeling a sense of purpose.
2. Plans and objectives, even if broad and general, are necessary pre-conditions to feeling a sense of achievement.
3. The broad Themes that lie behind specific objectives are more important than the individual objectives themselves.
4. The way we think about our Purpose, Plans and Objectives needs to be sufficiently robust and sufficiently flexible to cope with the events that life throws at us.

The rest of this chapter will help you to use a variety of approaches to create a personal set of Themes, Objectives and Plans that together will help you feel a sense of purpose. They will create the basis for feeling a sense of achievement, and will provide the basis for making decisions that fit with your Values. They will also help you recognise opportunities that come your way, and increase your ability to react in ways that make sense in the way you want to live. All of this is core to your personal contentment project.

## 4.3    Uncovering our built-in plans

The work that you did in creating the Values statements, ("I want to live my life on the basis of.....") will have created a strong picture of the sort of person you want to be, and probably the sort of person that to greater or lesser extent you already are. The exercises in the Values chapter were designed to help you gather evidence from your life about the Values that are driving your choices in time allocation and in decision making. They also should have helped identify what was lurking under the surface and was causing worry or sleeplessness. By the end of that chapter, the statements you wrote should have allowed you to make conscious choices about the Values that you want to have as the basis for how you live your life.

Human beings are complex organisms. We have the ability to use reasoning and logic to analyse and categorise before making rational decisions. However we also have intuition, gut feelings, and sub-conscious processes that are enormously important. If we make plans on the basis only of cold logic, our subconscious processes will catch up with us and will nag for attention. If we plan a direction that doesn't fit with some deeply held picture of who we are, there will be more sleeplessness and anxiety rather than less. So it is important to take this planning step on the basis of the "feelings" we have as well as on the basis of evidence-based analysis. The worksheets have been designed to combine these inputs, but the next stage is designed to focus much more clearly on the feelings and intuitions that are part of you.

Some counsellors talk about "scripts" that we carry with us. The script is rather like the screenplay for a movie, and once you are thoroughly immersed in it you are able to identify the characters and even predict how they are going to react to each event that hits them, and each decision they face. This is a graphic way of describing the influences that have formed the way we are. We react in ways that form patterns. I have yet to meet the individual whose responses to life were truly random. The pattern of responses is the outward manifestation of the script that we carry. The writing of that script is a fascinating process, as it involves both positive and negative reaction to the experiences we have. You will have used worksheets earlier to list your Heroes and Villains – the people you would like to emulate, as well as the people whose example you want to avoid. Generally we take on elements of our script without conscious thought. It is easier to observe this in others than it is to see it in ourselves. A very simple example is when you watch the child of a couple you know well, and you see the reflection in the child's behaviour of the parents' habits and preferences.

The positive thing about this is that we are not powerless viewers of the next instalment of the script. Rather like interactive television, we can influence the way the script develops. By reading this book and using the exercises as far as you already have, you have been interacting with your script. Things are not exactly the same as they were before you started.

The process that we are about to use is designed to uncover some of the built-in implications of the influences that you have experienced in your life. It is not looking at a logical analysis of the inputs, but looking at where that leaves you. What is the end product of all those influences on your life-script?

*Jack (who featured in previous examples) is a middle-aged, middle-class male, with the collection of worries, pressures and imperatives that drive many of us. His earlier exercises had led him to recognise the positive and negative influences on his current reactions. His father's energy, his mother's excessive politeness, Margaret Thatcher's views on society – all could be listed in his influences. He had clarified his thinking about his work-life balance, and made some preliminary resolutions. His statements about his Values seemed to be logical and sensible. He actually was quite happy with the six statements he had created. But he needed to take another perspective on them – to really stand back and get out of the detailed analysis so that he could see the "whole-life" picture, and allow all the key influences in his script to be checked against his work so far.*

*Jack's coach helped him to take a quiet time where he did something that at first seems a bit morbid. He challenged him to project himself forward beyond the end of his life, and to allow the combination of rational thought and intuitive feeling to guide him towards the obituary that he would be happy with. This very private exercise meant ignoring false modesty and trying to get on paper the big themes that for whatever reason he would like to see in his life. It only took a couple of hours, but it helped Jack to clarify and confirm the thoughts that had been emerging from the analysis. It created a word-picture that was a real insight for him, and summed up the features and histories that for whatever logical or "pre-programmed" reason he wanted to be present in his life. "I really would be unhappy if these things didn't feature in my life and if these things couldn't be said about me."*

The example of Jack's experience probably gives you almost enough guidance about the next exercise. You are asked to take a quiet time – at least an hour – to think and to commit to text the obituary that you would like someone to read following your death. The guidelines are as follows:

- Imagine an individual who knows you very well and has a good overview of your life. It can be a real person or an idealised combination of people.
- Use the perspective of this real or imagined person to write a short obituary for you.
- Think about what you would like to hear said about the "sort of person you were."
- Pick out the key things that you did that you would like to hear reported.
- Try to write the obituary in less than a page – probably only 3 or 4 paragraphs.
- Allow the big themes to come through. What would you be really sorry if they couldn't say about you by the end of your life?

This is a very personal and very thoughtful exercise. The last question is the most important. Allow it to bring to the surface whatever themes, achievements or descriptions that deep down inside you know you would like your friend to be able to read about you.

**Take time now to write the obituary before moving on to the next section.**

## 4.4    The sort of person I want to be:

That is a daunting title for the section.  It makes sense only if you have completed the previous exercises and have formed pictures about the key features that you can say you want to feature in your life.

Take time first to read some of the worksheets you have already produced.  The key items to look back over are:

- Chapter 2 – Summary of Strengths – especially the "Action" column
- Same chapter – History – especially the "What can I learn?" column
- Same chapter – Flip side – especially the "Well?" column
- Chapter 3 – your statements at the end of the chapter "I want to live my life on the basis of......"
- Chapter 4 (this chapter) – your obituary.

The review of all of these reflections will help you identify a list of "Themes" that you want to continue to pay attention to, and those you can see you need to pay more attention to.  You will find that the "I want to live my life on the basis of...." statements are the single most important input to the list of Themes, because they already synthesise the outcomes from your analysis.  But you will probably find that re-reading the other material, especially the obituary, will prompt one or two further Themes you want to build in.

Jack, our sample reviewer, used his Values statements to identify most of his themes, but adds two items.  One, he realises emerges from his Strengths and Flip Side review.  It is about the possibility of being less cold, logical and analytical all the time.  He identified that this strength of his had become inappropriate in some situations, but it was such an ingrained habit he needed to take positive steps to modify it. His obituary also had him thinking about the length of his life and a thought that frequently lurked but had not resulted in action was that he must do something about his health and fitness.

So Jack's list of Themes looked like this:

| Attention to family | Community contribution | Integrity | Friendship | Innovation | People rather than things | Relaxed and intuitive vs cold and logical | Health |
|---|---|---|---|---|---|---|---|

**Take time now to re-read the earlier worksheets and generate your list of Themes now.**

*Each one should be a short phrase or even a word that reminds you of the Theme that you are determined to build in to your life and your activities.*

| Themes | | | | | | | |
|---|---|---|---|---|---|---|---|
| | | | | | | | |

The next step is to list the broad areas of life where you can put this into practice. Jack has identified 5 aspects of his life that give him enough clarity. However you can choose more precise roles within those aspects of life. For example Jack has chosen simply "Work life" as an aspect.  You could equally well split that into several of the work roles you have – for example "Manager", "Colleague", "Expert".

Jack's sample is as follows:

| Aspect of life |
| --- |
| Family life |
| Work life |
| Friends |
| Spare time |
| Holidays |

Take time now to think about the aspects of life that will be useful for you to use when thinking about practical planning.  Try to have no fewer than 3 and no more than 8.

| Aspect of life |
| --- |
|  |
|  |
|  |
|  |
|  |
|  |
|  |
|  |

The next step is to plot the Themes against the Aspects of your life, to show in which part of your life you need to be doing something about the Theme you have identified.  Jack's example is shown below.  He has been able to identify that the key Aspect of his life where he needs to take some action on the "Attention to family" Theme is in his Work-life. He already pays attention to his family during his family time, and his holidays, but he knows that he needs to build in some attention to family in his work-life. Thinking about the impact on family of his business hours or his travel plans, would potentially pay off in allowing him to be more the sort of person he wants to be.

| Aspect \ Theme | Attention to family | Community comtribution | Integrity | Friendship | Innovation | People rather than things | Relaxed and intuitive vs cold and logical | Health |
|---|---|---|---|---|---|---|---|---|
| Family life | | | | | | ✓ | ✓ | |
| Work life | ✓ | | ✓ | | ✓ | | ✓ | |
| Friends | | | | ✓ | | | | |
| Spare time | ✓ | ✓ | | ✓ | | | | ✓ |
| Holidays | | | | | ✓ | | | |

Take time now to complete the following chart – inserting your list of Aspects of life; then listing the Themes you want to pay attention to; and finally ticking the boxes where you want to put the Theme into action. Try not to tick every box! You will make things manageable if you opt for between 6 and 12 ticks now. Next time you review the exercise you can add different ticks, but remember the old saying about "he who has too many priorities has no priorities!"

| | Theme | | | | | | | |
|---|---|---|---|---|---|---|---|---|
| **Aspect** | | | | | | | | |
| | | | | | | | | |
| | | | | | | | | |
| | | | | | | | | |
| | | | | | | | | |
| | | | | | | | | |

(Use this layout on your own full-size sheet of paper, or photocopy and enlarge the sample)

## 4.5    Setting Objectives

The matrix you have just completed gives the perfect basis for homing in on the practical plans that will make most difference in becoming the person you want to be.   It may be worth summarising the steps you have taken so far, as this is a long and thoughtful process.  Sometimes it is worthwhile to pause and look back over the path taken so far, as well as the steps still to come.

Contentment project

| Chapter | Section | Progress |
|---|---|---|
| Who I am | | |
| | My history | ✓ |
| | Strengths | ✓ |
| | Preferences | ✓ |
| | Dark side | ✓ |

| Chapter | Section | Progress |
|---|---|---|
| Values | | |
| | Time analysis | ✓ |
| | Decision analysis | ✓ |
| | Worry analysis | ✓ |
| | Influences | ✓ |
| | Values statements | ✓ |

| Chapter | Section | Progress |
|---|---|---|
| Purpose | | |
| | Identifying Themes | ✓ |
| | Identifying Aspects | ✓ |
| | Action matrix | ✓ |
| | Objectives and plans | |

| Chapter | Section | Progress |
|---|---|---|
| Relationships | | |
| | | |
| | | |

| Chapter | Section | Progress |
|---|---|---|
| Resources | | |
| | | |
| | | |

| Chapter | Section | Progress |
|---|---|---|
| Achievements | | |
| | | |
| | | |

As you can see, we are well on the way through the project, and the completion of the "Objectives and Plans" section completes the first 3 elements of the 6 core factors.

The layout that we are going to use allows for both short term action plans and longer term direction (stated as an objective).  For example, if like Jack you want to make some progress on the attention you pay to your family during your work-life, it is worth having both a broad general statement about where you want to get to, and also a short-term achievable target for the coming week.

Jack therefore needs a way of reminding himself of the overall direction he wants to take in the 12 boxes he ticked in the planning matrix, as well as a daily reminder of the practical action he can take.  This may sound laborious, but actually most of the hard work is already done, and you are now moving into the positive practical planning stage which is very rewarding!

The layout we are going to use is a paper-based one, but you will find it really helpful if you have a PDA or laptop that you can use to maintain your running objective sheet.  For each of the boxes you ticked in the planning matrix (hopefully no more than 12 and possibly only a smaller number) you will be creating:

- A statement of the long-term situation you want to achieve.  This will be a stable, long-term reminder of how things will be when you are demonstrating in one aspect of your life the Theme that you have chosen.

- A short term practical action that you can take, that will be a step in the right direction.  This will reflect what is happening in your life *this week and the next few weeks*, and will allow you to make the clear link between your overall direction and your day-to-day actions. While the long term statement probably should be reviewed only about once a year, the short-term action plans are a weekly cycle.

Step 1: Choose the first tick in your planning matrix and write in the "Objective" box below, the statement of how things will be when you are demonstrating that theme in the chosen aspect of your life. You have already carried out all the background analysis and thinking that you need to inform your statement, so try to quickly and briefly record the statement of "how things will be".

Step 2: Think about the week ahead, and identify at least one simple "achievable" action that will be a step in the right direction. Write this in the appropriate box.

A sample entry from Jack's plan is shown.

| Theme | Attention to family | | | Objective: | I will have achieved a balance in my work-life that allows me to be a successful and hard worker while giving time and attention to my family. I will no longer feel guilty about time allocation, and my family will be positive about my work and my time management. |
|---|---|---|---|---|---|
| Aspect | Work-life | | | | |

| | Item | Tick |
|---|---|---|
| Action: | Stop work by 6:00 pm on Friday | |
| | Check conference dates against family events | |
| | | |
| | | |
| | | |
| | | |
| | | |
| | | |
| | | |
| | | |

Note:

1. Jack has written in the Objective section a long-term objective, including a statement about how he will feel when he achieves this objective. This is by its nature going to take time to achieve, and probably will not be fully achieved in the coming year.

2. In the Action section, Jack has identified two simple achievable actions for the coming week. The first "Stop work by 6:00 pm on Friday," may well stay for a few weeks as a reminder, but once he has completed the second action it can be replaced by something that is relevant the following week. The key point is the immediacy and simplicity of the Actions. They relate to things you really can do in the coming week.

**Now fill in the following Objective and Action sheets for each of the boxes on the planning Matrix where you identified that you need to do something. Space is provided for six sets of objectives and actions.**

**(As before, you may find it best to create your own worksheets using the layout in the example)**

| Theme | | Objective: | |
|---|---|---|---|
| Aspect | | | |

| Action: | Item | Tick |
|---|---|---|
| | | |
| | | |
| | | |
| | | |
| | | |
| | | |
| | | |
| | | |
| | | |
| | | |

| Theme | | Objective: | |
|---|---|---|---|
| Aspect | | | |

| Action: | Item | Tick |
|---|---|---|
| | | |
| | | |
| | | |
| | | |
| | | |
| | | |
| | | |
| | | |
| | | |
| | | |

| Theme | | Objective: | |
|---|---|---|---|
| Aspect | | | |

| Action: | Item | Tick |
|---|---|---|
| | | |
| | | |
| | | |
| | | |
| | | |
| | | |
| | | |
| | | |
| | | |
| | | |

| Theme | | Objective: | |
|---|---|---|---|
| Aspect | | | |

| Action: | Item | Tick |
|---|---|---|
| | | |
| | | |
| | | |
| | | |
| | | |
| | | |
| | | |
| | | |
| | | |
| | | |
| | | |

| Theme | | Objective: | |
|---|---|---|---|
| Aspect | | | |

| Action: | Item | Tick |
|---|---|---|
| | | |
| | | |
| | | |
| | | |
| | | |
| | | |
| | | |
| | | |
| | | |
| | | |
| | | |

| Theme | | Objective: | |
|---|---|---|---|
| Aspect | | | |

| Action: | Item | Tick |
|---|---|---|
| | | |
| | | |
| | | |
| | | |
| | | |
| | | |
| | | |
| | | |
| | | |
| | | |
| | | |

Practical Hint:

You probably will not want to carry these planning sheets everywhere with you, but you can blend them into your personal style of task management. If you are a PDA user, you can choose which of the tasks should go on your task list. If you are a paper or back of an envelope user – list the few items you want to be able to tick off *today.* Whatever method you use, use the Objective and Task sheets as the basic management tool. Refer back to them to tick off completed tasks, and to choose today's tasks. Some people find it helpful to carry out the daily check at the end of the day, so that they can plan what will be on the list tomorrow. Others find it best to do it first thing in the morning. Choose a timing and method that feels right for you and that works for you.

# Chapter 5

# Satisfying relationships.

**Sections in Chapter 5**

# Chapter 5

## 5.1    Satisfying relationships

We seem to function or to have evolved in such a way that we need other people.  That isn't to say that we can't do without them - particularly for short periods of time - but the true recluse is the very rare exception.  For most purposes it seems that we operate best and are most content if we have the company of other people.

What works best for you will not be the same as the arrangement that works best for the person sitting next to you.  Individual differences, which come from our infinitely differing personalities and the unique learning we have accumulated over our lives, mean that it would be strange for there to be a universal formula that was the complete answer for all of us.  However there are guidelines and principles that you can apply to your own situation and personality.

Most people treat their relationships in ways that would lead to problems in any other area.  If I maintained my car as inadequately as I maintain some important relationships it would be dirty, unreliable and probably inoperative when I needed it most.  Thankfully good friends make more allowances than most cars.  But there are limits.

If you want to enjoy satisfying relationships you have to work on them and you have to manage them.  Managing them implies making a few decisions and sorting a few priorities.

There are 6 aspects that are easy to think about, and which you can use in a quick check of the way you are maintaining your relationships.

- *Number of relationships*
- *Groups of relationships*
- *Quality and depth*
- *Information flow*
- *Energy input*
- *Nuts and Bolts*

## 5.2    Number of relationships

There is an old saying that the person with lots of priorities has no priorities. To some extent the same can be said of relationships. People who concentrate on developing the greatest number of relationships will run the risk of making it difficult to put enough time into any one of them.

*Thomas is a successful professional, who is very good at striking up relationships with people. He is gifted in the way he can focus attention on someone and make them feel important and interesting. The lucky recipient of the attention can blossom and feel good about themselves for a while. Unfortunately the other side of the coin isn't long in turning up. He creates so many relationships that he automatically makes it impossible to avoid clashes of loyalty, difficulty finding time to meet, and ultimately he causes bad feeling and disillusionment. The person who has been seduced into feeling that they are the new "best friend" soon feels rejection and disappointment when they inevitably see the same level of attention and encouragement lavished on someone else. Over time, the reality of the situation becomes clear. Thomas knows where he is going wrong, but is so busy being successful that he is putting off the day when he decides to invest in really sound relationships.*

The message that a new person meeting Thomas receives may be,

*"On the basis of the attention I paying to you, the empathetic way I'm responding to you, the obvious respect and fascination I feel for you, I am immediately making you a very important person in my world, and admitting you to my inner circle of important friends."*

The reality behind the scene is actually that Thomas is thinking,

*"I'm so skilled at this. I really have this person eating out of my hand. My body-language and eye-contact are spot-on in conveying interest and attention. This really is interesting, and this person could be a useful contact, but I had better remember to pick up those e-mails and get back to the office in good time."*

Skill and artifice can be wonderful at quickly establishing contact, but they don't form the basis for a satisfying, honest and long-lasting relationship. There is a danger for those who have developed high skills in this area that they unthinkingly seduce people into what is essentially a false relationship. Those lacking skills in relating, face the opposite problem of failing to develop what could be good relationships, and wonder why.

More crucial than your level of skill is your honesty of intention. However if you know that your level of skill in relating to people is a handicap - it is probably worth investing some time in improving it. Most local libraries will have a list of courses and workshops that can help. If you can't find a course specifically on developing relationships, join a practical course or group where you will have to relate to others – choose something interesting and stimulating – the relationships will follow.

It is easiest to be honest in your intention if you have some easy way of thinking about the range of relationships that are manageable.
Think in terms of concentric circles:

The inner circle is ME.

The dark inner circle contains my warmest closest friends. (How many can I "maintain" in this circle?)

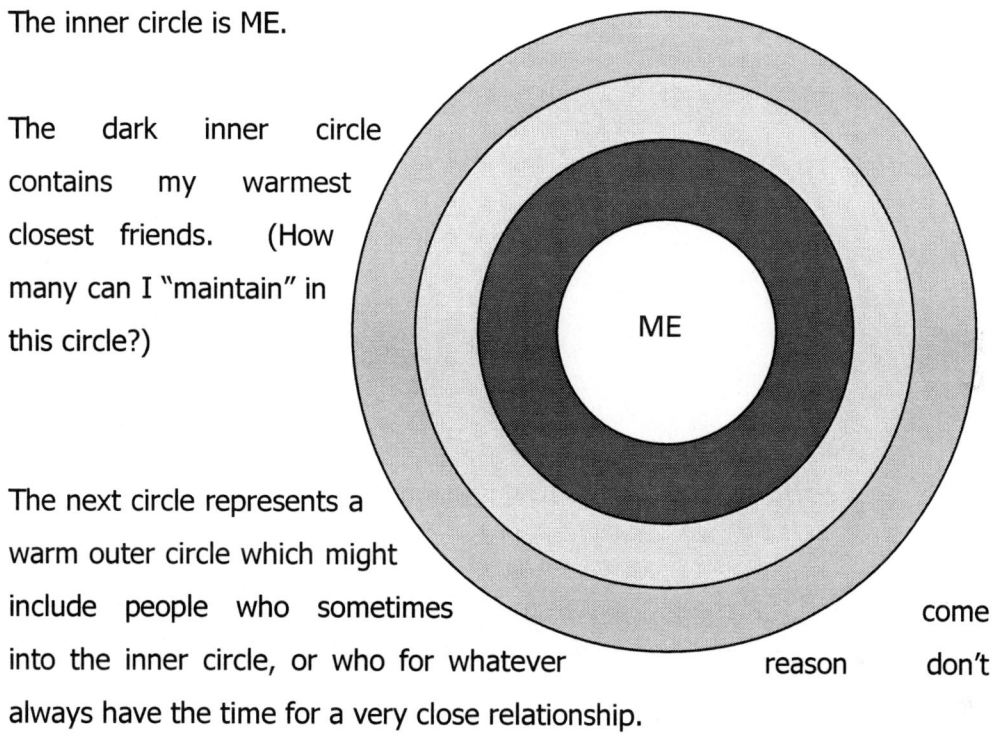

The next circle represents a warm outer circle which might include people who sometimes come into the inner circle, or who for whatever reason don't always have the time for a very close relationship.

The outer circle is for the wider range of acquaintances – greater in number, great to have, but different in demand and time-consumption from the inner circle.

The lines between the circles are not necessarily permanent – people can move from one to another, but it helps to make appropriate decisions about allocation of time and attention if you can think in terms of some differentiations. An inner circle friend can expect more time and a greater readiness on my part to drop other concerns when they need me.  If I try to treat everyone on that basis I end up unable to practise a really close relationship with anyone.

## 5.3    Groups of relationships – the three-legged stool:

Observation of many people and situations over the years suggests that the three-legged stool principle is relevant.    It is rare for people to experience just one main relationship or set of relationships.  Most of us have at least two main sets of relationships - for example a spouse at home and a set of work colleagues.  It is more common again for people to have greater numbers of sets of relationships.  It is clear that a minimum of three different types of relationship helps to keep us balanced and is more likely to be conducive to feelings of contentment.

### Variety is the spice:

The couple who relate only to each other and their immediate family become disconnected from the rest of life.  Their judgement becomes uncertain, as they know how limited their contacts are, and they lack the confidence that comes from healthy exchange and testing of ideas with other types of people.

Even for those who have found their "soul-mate", the relationship works best in the context of other relationships.  Apart from a brief honeymoon period the relationship that exists without wider contacts quickly becomes stifling, frustrating and negative.

The classic "opposition" of home and work is similar.  Have you met people who have no relationships other than family outside of work?  They are often literally two-dimensional characters. Conversation tends to be limited; interest in external affairs similarly so; and crucially from a business as well as a personal well-being point of view, their perspective suffers. They usually are so wrapped up in their world of work that they don't have any capacity for standing outside the situation and taking a balanced view of issues. They can often be the people who make mountains out of minor issues, take offence where none was intended, and have more difficulty than others in coping well with problems and difficulties at work.

In contrast, picture the colleague who comes to work having been mentally recharged through some totally unrelated but stimulating external hobby or interest. It might be an evening of activity and conversation in their club. It might be the amateur artist who has spent time learning with friends how to achieve the perfect colour combination for their latest watercolour, or the bowler who has enjoyed an evening of competition and laughter. They are much more likely to be able to take a balanced view of problems and annoyances. They achieve a different perspective because other contacts have of necessity dragged them away from being wrapped up in one set of concerns. You can choose for yourself which seems more healthy, and more likely to be helpful in achieving contentment.

*This leads us back to the proposition that a minimum of THREE sets of relationships is the requirement that most of us experience.*

That might mean any combination of a spouse/partner; a set of work colleagues; and friends in a club or class. It might equally be the combined set of home relationships, the people you meet in Church, and the friends in the painting class you attend.

The key requirement is the variety of the nature of relationships. The young man whose relationships are all variations on the theme of drinking companions in different settings will quickly become a limited and limiting companion. As will the devout Church supporter or political activist whose relationships are all within that context.

The successful executive whose friendships are limited to other successful executives - no matter how many - will suffer similar limitations in outlook and in their feelings of contentment.

**Exercise:**

Draw on the next page a diagram of the frequent and important relationships you have. List the people - grouping them where appropriate.

See if you can circle the groups that fit into a similar category for whatever reason.

Ask yourself if you have your "3-legged stool" - with sufficient variety and interest to keep you stimulated and contented.

*Simplified sample drawing:*

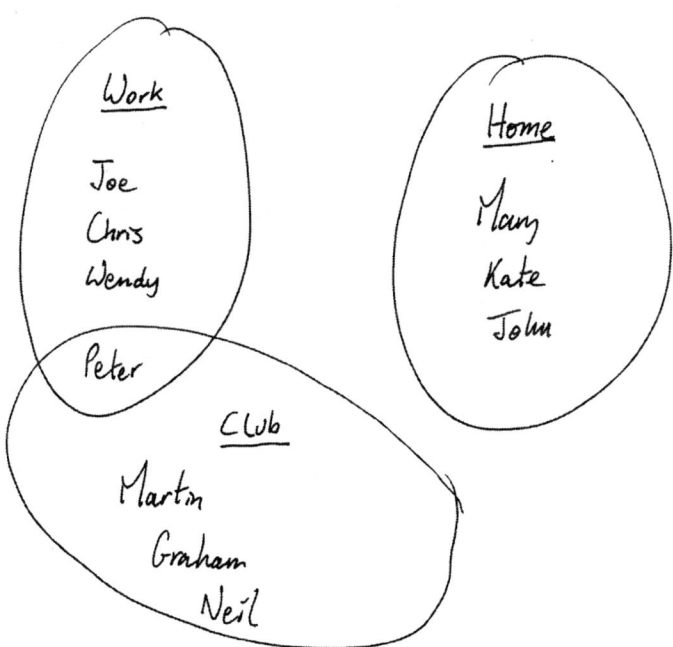

In this example, there is an overlap between Work and Club. Is this helpful do you think? There is a danger that issues and worries from one arena will interfere with the other. It depends in this case on how Peter handles it, and how I handle it - but it could ruin the club as a separate leg of the stool!

Your Drawing:

## 5.4    Quality and depth of relationship

Think about the relationships that have lasted well for you.  What are the characteristics that set those relationships apart from the more superficial and less satisfying relationships?

What quality of relationship do you want?  Are you clear about the implications of that for the depth of relationship that you need to work towards?  Are you prepared to make the investments that are needed to make it a real "inner circle" relationship?

These include:

- Revealing more of your self and your feelings than you may be used to doing
- Seeking as much information and insight as you give.
- Accepting the need sometimes to act as a counsellor to the other, and working hard at listening and questioning.
- Making time for maintaining the relationship
- Keeping confidential the bits of information you would love to share with others
- Maintaining a high level of honesty and open-ness
- Being thoughtful beforehand, and remembering to share things of interest to the other.

Use the following self-rating scale to assess the extent to which your relationships live up to your aspiration for them.  Use the "Action" column to tick the items that you know you need to do something about.  These will be gathered later for action planning. .

| Friend "a" | V Low | | Low | | Average | | High | | V High | | Action? |
|---|---|---|---|---|---|---|---|---|---|---|---|
| | 1 | 2 | 3 | 4 | 5 | 6 | 7 | 8 | 9 | 10 | |
| Revealing more of your self and your feelings | | | | | | | | | | | |
| Seeking information | | | | | | | | | | | |
| Working hard at listening and questioning | | | | | | | | | | | |
| Making time | | | | | | | | | | | |
| Keeping confidential | | | | | | | | | | | |
| Honesty and open-ness | | | | | | | | | | | |
| Being thoughtful beforehand | | | | | | | | | | | |

| Friend "b" | V Low | | Low | | Average | | High | | V High | | Action? |
|---|---|---|---|---|---|---|---|---|---|---|---|
| | 1 | 2 | 3 | 4 | 5 | 6 | 7 | 8 | 9 | 10 | |
| Revealing more of your self and your feelings | | | | | | | | | | | |
| Seeking information | | | | | | | | | | | |
| Working hard at listening and questioning | | | | | | | | | | | |
| Making time | | | | | | | | | | | |
| Keeping confidential | | | | | | | | | | | |
| Honesty and open-ness | | | | | | | | | | | |
| Being thoughtful beforehand | | | | | | | | | | | |

| Friend "c" | V Low | | Low | | Average | | High | | V High | | Action? |
|---|---|---|---|---|---|---|---|---|---|---|---|
| | 1 | 2 | 3 | 4 | 5 | 6 | 7 | 8 | 9 | 10 | |
| Revealing more of your self and your feelings | | | | | | | | | | | |
| Seeking information | | | | | | | | | | | |
| Working hard at listening and questioning | | | | | | | | | | | |
| Making time | | | | | | | | | | | |
| Keeping confidential | | | | | | | | | | | |
| Honesty and open-ness | | | | | | | | | | | |
| Being thoughtful beforehand | | | | | | | | | | | |

| Friend "d" | V Low | | Low | | Average | | High | | V High | | Action? |
|---|---|---|---|---|---|---|---|---|---|---|---|
| | 1 | 2 | 3 | 4 | 5 | 6 | 7 | 8 | 9 | 10 | |
| Revealing more of your self and your feelings | | | | | | | | | | | |
| Seeking information | | | | | | | | | | | |
| Working hard at listening and questioning | | | | | | | | | | | |
| Making time | | | | | | | | | | | |
| Keeping confidential | | | | | | | | | | | |
| Honesty and open-ness | | | | | | | | | | | |
| Being thoughtful beforehand | | | | | | | | | | | |

# Notes of action items to remember:

## 5.5    Information flow

When you are relating to people that you would like to have in your "inner circle", take a note of the direction of the flow of information.  Are you on the receiving end of a long catalogue of the activities, successes, disasters or ailments of the other person?  Are they perhaps on the receiving end of your no-doubt fascinating input?

The best relationships almost certainly have a balance of information flow over time.  On some occasions it is natural for one person to have more to report of their activities or problems.  But if you find yourself always listening and not being asked about your life, you will find the relationship unsettling and unhelpful.

> *Joan is a hard-working business owner.  She is fully occupied with work and with home life, but knows that she needs to take time to keep relationships alive and functioning.  She tries to meet each of her inner circle friends every month, but finds herself putting off contacting one of them.  When questioned in detail about the relationship, Joan realises that the reason she puts off this contact is that she finds it is more of a duty than a pleasure.  When we track the flow of information in a typical lunch-time chat, we find that Joan does a lot of listening, a lot of reacting to the news she is receiving from her friend, and quite a lot of follow-up questioning.  What is not happening is her friend demonstrating interest in Joan's life.  She is not asking about Joan's family, work, or problems.*

This is a problem that seems to affect many people who are professionally skilled in relating to others.  They have learned through work to demonstrate interest, and to be effective in asking questions. What they need is for others to demonstrate similar levels of skill in relating to them. If you need a friend to change, perhaps it is time for you to use your skills in giving some constructive feedback to your friend. You might even share the following diagnosis with them.

**Information flow diagnosis:**

Is this you?

"You are conscious that you do most of the talking, but that is because you are the noisy one, and you have an interesting life that your friends are always glad to hear about."

Are you sure? Next time you have lunch with a friend, do the following review afterwards:

| Question | Well? | Action? |
|---|---|---|
| What percentage of the time did you spend giving information or opinions? If it was honestly more than about 70% ask yourself if this is usual, or just because you had a lot to tell on this occasion? | | |
| What can you remember of the things that your friend said? | | |
| What was their news? | | |
| What is worrying them today? | | |
| How many questions did you ask? | | |

## 5.6    Energy input

This is somewhat similar to the question of Information Flow.  We all adopt a pattern in the amount of energy we put into relationships.  It happens whether we think about it or not.  Some of us become the reactive partners in most of our relationships.  Some by nature are more likely to take initiatives.  However this is one pattern that is absolutely within our power to change.  With a little thought we can decide if we need to put more energy into relationships, and if so, which ones.

On the following worksheet you are asked to rate the level of your energy input with each of four friends.  Photocopy the page if necessary to include other people.  The headings you are rating yourself on are as follows:

- Likely to suggest meeting.  - *Honestly assess the extent to which you are the one to suggest getting together.  An average rating means you are doing only as well as most other people.  A high rating means that you are playing your full part – not necessarily that you are always the one to suggest meeting.  It is possible for two friends both to score high in this.*

- Taking initiatives about location or time  - *This should be easy to remember.  Are you the one who passively goes along with suggestions?  Do you put effort into thinking about what would be stimulating, or the location that would be most convenient?*

- Putting energy into questioning, probing  - *This should reflect your answer in the "information flow" section.  Do you ask follow-up questions? Are you probing behind the surface story? Are you asking "how do you really feel about that"?*

- Energetic listening  - . *Are you demonstrating genuine active interest in what your friend is saying.  If I were to observe you would you be making eye contact and looking interested. Would I see you reacting to what you are hearing? Are you able to recall well what information or stories your friend conveyed?*

- Keeping up contact - *Apart from contact to set up a meeting, do you ring to see how things are going? Do you forward interesting e-mails? Do you send texts about tv programmes your friend might like to see?*

- Following up "matters arising" - *When you say "I must send you a copy of that article," do you do it? Do you find yourself later noticing something that relates to your conversation and taking action to mention it to your friend? When you agree that it would be a good idea to organise something are you the one to follow up?*

When you have completed the self-rating chart, allow yourself some time for reflection. You may well want to complete the ratings for more than the 4 friends listed on the sheet, so make copies if you need to. Be as honest as you can in rating yourself – neither unnecessarily harsh nor easy. When you have filled in your answers take time to look at the picture that emerges and ask yourself if it looks right. There is a small space for "Notes" after the rating. It is deliberately small so you don't think of a million things to change.

- Who are the people or who is the person with whom you should change the energy input? Maybe you are putting in too much energy with one person and not enough with others? Are real "inner circle" friends getting enough energy from you?
- Can you make a short checklist of things to do if actions are needed?

- If it looks about right allow yourself a little self-recognition for a job well done!

# Self-rating of Energy input to relationships

**My input with:**
**Friend "a"**

| | V Low | | Low | | Average | | High | | V High | | Action? |
|---|---|---|---|---|---|---|---|---|---|---|---|
| | 1 | 2 | 3 | 4 | 5 | 6 | 7 | 8 | 9 | 10 | |
| Likely to suggest meeting | | | | | | | | | | | |
| Taking initiatives about location or time | | | | | | | | | | | |
| Putting energy into questioning, probing | | | | | | | | | | | |
| Energetic listening | | | | | | | | | | | |
| Keeping up contact | | | | | | | | | | | |
| Following up "matters arising" | | | | | | | | | | | |

**My input with:**
**Friend "b"**

| | V Low | | Low | | Average | | High | | V High | | Action? |
|---|---|---|---|---|---|---|---|---|---|---|---|
| | 1 | 2 | 3 | 4 | 5 | 6 | 7 | 8 | 9 | 10 | |
| Likely to suggest meeting | | | | | | | | | | | |
| Taking initiatives about location or time | | | | | | | | | | | |
| Putting energy into questioning, probing | | | | | | | | | | | |
| Energetic listening | | | | | | | | | | | |
| Keeping up contact | | | | | | | | | | | |
| Following up "matters arising" | | | | | | | | | | | |

**My input with:**
**Friend "c"**

| | V Low | | Low | | Average | | High | | V High | | Action? |
|---|---|---|---|---|---|---|---|---|---|---|---|
| | 1 | 2 | 3 | 4 | 5 | 6 | 7 | 8 | 9 | 10 | |
| Likely to suggest meeting | | | | | | | | | | | |
| Taking initiatives about location or time | | | | | | | | | | | |
| Putting energy into questioning, probing | | | | | | | | | | | |
| Energetic listening | | | | | | | | | | | |
| Keeping up contact | | | | | | | | | | | |
| Following up "matters arising" | | | | | | | | | | | |

**My input with:**
**Friend "d"**

| | V Low | | Low | | Average | | High | | V High | | Action? |
|---|---|---|---|---|---|---|---|---|---|---|---|
| | 1 | 2 | 3 | 4 | 5 | 6 | 7 | 8 | 9 | 10 | |
| Likely to suggest meeting | | | | | | | | | | | |
| Taking initiatives about location or time | | | | | | | | | | | |
| Putting energy into questioning, probing | | | | | | | | | | | |
| Energetic listening | | | | | | | | | | | |
| Keeping up contact | | | | | | | | | | | |
| Following up "matters arising" | | | | | | | | | | | |

## 5.7    Nuts and Bolts

Even when we have all the best intentions in the world, it is perfectly possible for things not to happen.  The "nuts and bolts" list is designed to be a gentle thought-provoker, to help you identify those simple things you could do that would help make it all work in practice.  Lots of them are simple almost routine things that we take for granted.  Some just help make it possible to manage a relationship better.

Use the following headings to reflect on the way you manage your relationships, and take time to make notes on the things you would like to do differently.  They may not be things that you are doing badly – it may just be time to try a change.

**Time for relationships:**

Observe what actually happens rather than what you would ideally like to happen.  How much time did you give last week to maintaining healthy relationships?  How much time this week?  No-matter what your theoretical position on maintaining relationships, this very simple measure will give you a no-nonsense piece of data on the importance you really give the issue.

You can count the time spent on telephone calls, e-mailing, and writing as well as the time spent actually meeting.  Try to differentiate between the relationships that, while friendly, are really for work or professional purposes.  Concentrate on those that you would see as important outside the work or professional context.

**Pattern of meeting:**

You probably have very different patterns of meeting for different people. Some relationships are based on quite infrequent activity. Others need much more constant care. Some are helped by routines that mean you don't have to think about organising a get-together, it happens because of natural circumstances – like the friend you meet every month after a club committee meeting.

The challenge is to check over each of the patterns and make sure that they make sense. Try to identify any that are languishing because you don't get together sufficiently frequently. Identify also those that get too much of your time and attention. Don't forget you can manage your time. It is precious, and it is very easy to allow habits to carry on when they are no longer needed.

**Variety of contact:**

Think about your range of contact methods. Most of us will list face-to-face meetings, telephone, e-mail and texting. Do you use all of them with the people who most appreciate them? Can you think up alternatives that would inject some novelty into the relationship? What about the occasional hand-written letter? What about picture post-cards that take only a moment to send? What about inexpensive gifts from time to time that show you have thought about the person?

See if you can think of at least one variation on your usual pattern that would inject some positive new life into a relationship.

## Location and setting:

When you do meet fact to face, are you using the choice of setting as a positive bonus?  You can probably identify the friends for whom a lively, noisy café is perfect.  There are others who need somewhere more restful and less challenging.  There may be periods in relationships where there are sensitive issues to be talked about – when privacy is important.  There may be people who need to be given a little pzazz, others who need time for quiet chat and even for long pauses without chat.  Are there people for whom it is better to meet while having a long walk?

Think through all your usual habits and try to identify one example of a change that would be helpful to the relationship.  The person who you always meet for a pub lunch might find an hour's walk a refreshing change.  The get-together that is always rushed might benefit from a long lazy dinner.

## Organising your data:

This may sound too organised for some people!  However it is so much easier for you to manage your friendships if you have your data organised.  Can you find all the relevant phone numbers easily?  The answer to that is generally "yes", as cell phone memories make up for our deficiencies.  But is the data available elsewhere when you lose your phone?  Do you have a backed-up set of electronic data that means you will not be too devastated by the loss of your phone, the theft of your filofax, or the crash of your PDA?

While you are organising the data – make sure that you make life easier for yourself.  If you use any of the mainstream address-book software you will be able to include all those bits of information that it is embarrassing to forget:  names of family, birthdays and anniversaries are probably the most important, but use the technology to help you. You can categorise people in your contact list. Label those you want to remember to send a Christmas card, New Year's card or whatever you like to celebrate. You can easily then sort the list and print it out. Create groups in your e-mail contacts so that you can easily send an update to all those involved in a group activity.

## 5.8    Self review:

Use the table below to record your self-assessment on each of those items and the action points that you want to remember.

| Item | Self-assessment: How am I doing? | Action: What would be useful or positive to try? |
|---|---|---|
| Time given to relationships. | | |
| Pattern of contact. | | |
| Variety of contact methods. | | |
| Location and setting. | | |
| Organising data. | | |

# Chapter 6

# Resources

**Sections in Chapter 6**

Section 6.1   Why are resources important?

Section 6.2   Resource list examples

Section 6.3   Resources warm-up exercise

Section 6.4   Resource planner

Section 6.5   Next step – link back to action plans

Section 6.6   Review

# Chapter 6

# Resources

## 6.1 Why are resources important?

You have now completed most of the analytical aspects of your Contentment Project and are ready to make progress with your weekly action plans. The action plans will help you work your way towards the long term objectives that you have established.

The chapter on Purpose and Objectives highlighted the potential for "Events" – the things that happen day by day – to derail the best laid plans. Hopefully you have been able to use the combination of clear long term objectives and flexible short term plans to remain able to react to change. This will also help you recognise and respond to opportunities that fit in with your overall objective, even though you had not planned for them.

The other issue that needs to be addressed is that of Resources. Do not fall into the trap of feeling disabled by lack of resources. "If I had the money I could......"! In fact as you work through this chapter you will find that most of the resources you need are probably things that you have or that you can change. Realism is essential of course. It is not helpful to finding contentment if we plan activities that require resources that we cannot reasonably expect to have. However you may be surprised to find that most of the resources you need are things that you can control.

This chapter will help you think in a broader than usual way about the resources that you can make use of. We will cover:

- Your personal resources including the strengths you have already identified
  - Mental (including know-how)
  - Physical (including health, and skills)
  - Emotional
  - Social/interpersonal
  - Organisational
- People who can be helpful
- The material resources you have
- The local resources you can access
- Time
- Money

This chapter will help you remind yourself of the resources you can call on to help you achieve the weekly action plans, and to help you move towards the long-term objectives you have set. In some cases you will find a virtuous circle, where you may need to plan to increase one of your resources, and this becomes part of your action-planning. For example, if you plan to read about a topic that interests you, joining the local library could be an early action plan. Once you have ticked off that task you are creating the positive feeling of achievement that comes through each of the little steps that you take towards the long term objective.

The good thing about how we react is that even small steps in the right direction can have enormously beneficial effects on our feeling of achievement, of progress, and of contentment. We achieve feelings of contentment when we sense movement towards our long term objectives, not just when we get there. That is an enormously valuable bonus in the process, as most of us might give up if we had to wait for the final achievement before we experienced any reward.

The thought process we will go through in this chapter involves creating an inventory using the headings listed above.  You will do this in the context of your Objectives and Action Plans so that you identify where the resources can help.  You will also be able to identify where you need to do something to increase a resource, or make it more readily available.  You will then add the item to your action plan.

Some resources will be broadly useful across the whole set of tasks, but some may be specific to one or two tasks.  You will find it rewarding to create tasks that provide the resource you need – because they will often unlock the process of achieving the main objective.

Take the first of your objectives.  Jack's example is that of adjusting his work-life to allow him to give the time he wants to the family.  His simple task list includes only two items to start with – stopping work by 6:00 pm on Friday, and checking conference and meeting dates against family event dates.   Jack can identify when pushed that there are actually very useful things he can do when he thinks about the resources that are available.

First of all when he thinks about what keeps him late at the office on Fridays, it is a combination of tidying up at the end of the week and discussing the week's issues with a couple of his colleagues.  Neither of the colleagues has family ties.  They will be either going out socialising later on Friday evening, or having an evening alone at home.  Neither is in a great rush to leave the office before 7:00 pm.  Jack realises that his colleagues are part of the solution, just as they are part of the problem.  It isn't their fault that he stays late, but without their help it will be harder for him to break the habit.  So he lists the two colleagues as "people who can help", and makes a plan to explain to them what he is trying to do.  What happens here is a virtuous circle – because the identification of the need to talk to his colleagues about his plan not only helps solve the problem, but also makes it much more likely that he will be able to achieve his new action plan target of getting home at 6:00 pm on Fridays.

Jack's original action plan:

| Theme | Attention to family | | Objective: | I will have achieved a balance in my work-life that allows me to be a successful and hard worker while giving time and attention to my family. I will no longer feel guilty about time allocation, and my family will be positive about my work and my time management. |
|---|---|---|---|---|
| Aspect | Work-life | | | |

| | Item | Tick |
|---|---|---|
| Action: | Stop work by 6:00 pm on Friday | |
| | Check conference dates against family events | |
| | | |
| | | |
| | | |
| | | |
| | | |
| | | |
| | | |
| | | |

*Jack's resource identification prompts an extra action item which will make his first action attainable.*

## Sample first lines of Resource Planning Sheet:

| | Objective: | |
|---|---|---|
| **Summary:** *I will have achieved a balance in my work-life* | | |

| | Item | Resources |
|---|---|---|
| **Action:** | Stop work by 6:00 pm on Friday | Colleagues - Trish and John<br><br>Personal strength - determination |
| | Check conference dates against family events | Computer diaries for home and office |

*Jack's Action Plan now looks like this with the extra Action added:*

| | | | |
|---|---|---|---|
| **Theme** | **Attention to family** | **Objective:** | I will have achieved a balance in my work-life that allows me to be a successful and hard worker while giving time and attention to my family. I will no longer feel guilty about time allocation, and my family will be positive about my work and my time management. |
| **Aspect** | **Work-life** | | |

| | Item | Tick |
|---|---|---|
| **Action:** | Stop work by 6:00 pm on Friday | |
| | Check conference dates against family events | |
| | Explain Friday 6:00 pm plan to Trish and John and agree how we do it. | |
| | | |
| | | |
| | | |
| | | |
| | | |
| | | |

## 6.2    Resource list examples

Next step is to identify the resources that will be useful – to get the brain warmed up first complete the warm-up exercise.  The following are prompts and thought-starters rather than comprehensive lists – so use them as a springboard rather than a constraint.

## Resource examples

### Mental (including know-how)

Think of all the strengths you identified in the "Who am I" chapter worksheets. There will be things you are good at – that people assume you will be able to do. They may be to do with the way you think, be it analytically or imaginatively. Both are strengths although they are very different. You may have technical know-how that will be useful. Your computer skills, or your ability to write good letters may be worth listing. If you do not see yourself as academic, recognise that you have strengths in your practical and realistic analysis of issues. Conversely if you do not think you are practical and realistic, are you good at abstract or imaginative "big-picture" thinking?

### Physical (including health and skills)

Some of your strengths may be quite literally physical strength or ability. Think also of the skills that you have developed, whether at work or in your hobbies. We take for granted some of the health and wellbeing we enjoy. If health is a problem for you, this may be a very important area for sorting an objective and some action plans if you have not already done so. You will have been exposed to plenty of newspaper articles and television programmes about the extent to which exercise affects feelings of wellbeing. However it is hard to over-emphasise how important this is. Physical exercise does more than keep muscles in tone.  Very importantly it also affects the chemical balance of our bodies, and this affects our mood and our sense of well-being.  If you have issues about exercise and health, don't duck them.  This is important, as it has impact on every aspect of your feeling of being able to achieve your goals, and on your level of contentment.  It will be the exceptional person who does not need to have some sort of objective relating to health and physical exercise in their plan.

## Emotional

Look back again to the worksheets where you identified your strengths.  Your emotional resources will be different from mine.  One person's patience and tolerance can be their strength just as much as someone else's impatience and energy can be theirs.  Self-confidence may be one person's strength, while their counterpart has a strength in always questioning themselves.  There are two sides to all of these emotional features we enjoy (or perhaps suffer from!).  Don't do yourself down, but see the realistic features of your personality as resources that you need to use.

## Social/interpersonal

You may have identified your ability to create relationships as a strength – or quite the opposite.  Think again about those strengths you have in this area.  Are they about listening, or perhaps about expressing yourself to others.  We often see the gifted speaker as a good communicator, but the gifted listener may be a better learner, and may find it easier to make progress on their contentment project.  Be realistic about the strengths you have, and if there is something you need to do to develop greater strengths, make sure this is reflected in your Objectives and your Task planning.

## Organisational

Back again to your Strengths analysis.  Think about the things you identified that you were good at – whether they were in the Strategy/planning, the Operational or the IT/paper sections.  Strengths in this section can be doubly useful in helping you organise yourself in your Contentment Project, and in making sure that you put plans into action.  So take time to think back to your strengths and to recognise what will be useful, and also to identify if there are organisational strengths you need to develop.  If there are, you may need to include them in your Action Plans.

## People who can be helpful

Some of the people you will identify will be very specific to the objective and task in your plan.  For example Jack identified Trish and John as people who could help with one specific aspect of his plan.  There will be others who can help with your general thinking and planning.  The key point is that you shouldn't be reluctant to think of people as potential helpers.  Most of them will be flattered and energised by being used in some way.  People love to be involved in something purposeful. They also love to feel important and useful to someone else.  You really may make someone's day by asking for their help!  So don't be reluctant to think about this resource.

## Material resources

Look around you. You are looking at material resources – whether it is the room you are sitting in, the house you are living in, the computer in the spare room, or the books in your bedroom. You may have material resources that you are not using well at present. For example there may be a space you could use to think and write – but you need to clear it. There may be a family computer that you could learn to use more effectively. The internet access you have may be useful – think about upgrading it if it isn't easy and fast to use. What about your phone, your car, your garden? If you have them – are you able to use them helpfully? This is a two-way process. You are both identifying things you already have that will be useful resources, and also identifying things that you may need to change if they are going to be useful. Change doesn't necessarily mean spending money! Clearing a space and creating an area that you like to work in may simply require a bit of effort. It would create a Task for your plan that will be satisfying to complete, and that will in turn make it easier to achieve many of your other tasks.

Make sure that you do have that work-space. It might be the kitchen table in the evening, or it might be a desk in the study. If you are going to work on your Contentment Project you need to be able to think, write, organise and manage yourself. If you feel that your work area is a mess, your project will be that bit harder to implement. If you are organised in a way that suits you, things will happen more easily.

## Local Resources

You may have already identified some key local resources in the "people who can help". But think also about the local physical resources. The library is an obvious possibility for access to information and research. If physical health and fitness are part of your action planning, the gym will be useful. Don't forget the out-door resources. I should remember the mountains and the coastal path that are not far away which provide just as important a resource as the gym that I go to.

If your action plan involves developing yourself in some way – and it is almost certain that it does – think about the local groups that exist to support that interest. Whether it is the development of new skills, or pursuing a new interest, you may find classes, clubs and people that will help you on your way.

## Time

The finite resource! You may excuse yourself from not taking action because you do not have time. This is probably the most universal reason that we humans use for not doing the things that we leave undone. It is also one of the easiest to do something about. Your job or your family duties may mean that some times of the day you would find it really hard to make yourself available for a new project. For a large part of my working life I have been required to travel so much that joining a group that met on a specific week-night was simply impossible. I could never guarantee that I would be there. However that didn't mean that I didn't have time to do something useful. My failure to do so was usually down to me.

Think of the patterns of your days and imagine the changes you could make if you wanted to. For many people television is the single biggest factor in the time problem. If you genuinely do not spend any time watching things that are "optional", then you are in a very small minority. Most people could create some useful time for other activities if they changed their television routine.

Think also of the times of the day. Could you create some time by going to bed earlier and getting up earlier? Some people find that an hour in the morning before the rest of the world is bothering them is worth its weight in gold. You don't have to do it forever. Would it be worth trying for 6 months?

When you think of Time, think creatively. It may seem finite but it is enormously flexible, and human beings have great skill in manipulating it to create time for the things they really want to do. To enjoy contentment, you need to be satisfied that you are using your time in the way you want to. This does not mean super-human levels of activity. It may mean ensuring that you have time for real rest and reflection.

## Money

Finally "money"! The second most frequent excuse people use for not doing things that they suspect they should be doing. This is surprisingly the item that you should spend least time on. It is likely to be the least important. Just for the warm-up exercise, think of a few examples of money that you currently spend that you do not really need to (it might be as simple as the Sunday paper that you could give up for a time). Don't waste time on this, but when you work through each of your Objectives and Action Plans, be ruthlessly honest about the resources you really need to make them happen.

Your personal resources in terms of determination, motivation, thinking and organisation are likely to be far more important than money.

**Now complete the warm-up exercise.**

## 6.3    Resources Warm-up Exercise

Limit yourself to three examples in each category, but do try to list 3.

| Resource | 3 Examples |
|---|---|
| *Personal* | |
| • Mental (including know-how) | •<br><br>•<br><br>• |
| • Physical (including health and skills) | •<br><br>•<br><br>• |
| • Emotional | •<br><br>•<br><br>• |
| • Social/interpersonal | •<br><br>•<br><br>• |
| • Organisational | •<br><br>•<br><br>• |

| *External* | |
|---|---|
| • People who can be helpful | • <br><br> • <br><br> • |
| • Material resources | • <br><br> • <br><br> • |
| • Local resources | • <br><br> • <br><br> • |
| • Time | • <br><br> • <br><br> • |
| • Money | • <br><br> • <br><br> • |

## 6.4    Resource Planner

Now use the Resource Planner on page 144 to identify the relevant resources for each of your objectives:  Copy this sheet for each of your main objectives (probably 6 – 12).  Don't be intimidated by the number of spaces for actions! To start you will probably only have the first couple of lines completed, but over a few months you will work your way down the sheet.

- Write a phrase or sentence that summarises the objective (if it is too long to fit easily).
- Write in the action items you have already identified.
- List the first one or two resources you need

*See Jack's example from page 133*

| Objective: | |
|---|---|
| **Summary:** *I will have achieved a balance in my work-life* | |

| | Item | Resources |
|---|---|---|
| **Action:** | Stop work by 6:00 pm on Friday | Colleagues - Trish and John |
| | | Personal strength - determination |
| | Check conference dates against family events | Computer diaries for home and office |

## 6.5    Next step:   (After completing the Resource Planning sheets)

Make sure that you have made the link from the resources you have identified back to your Action Plans.  Review each of your 6 – 12 Objective sheets and check that you have written down the actions that were prompted by the thinking about resources.

| Objective: | | |
|---|---|---|
| **Summary:** | | |

| | Item | Resources |
|---|---|---|
| **Action:** | | |
| | | |
| | | |
| | | |
| | | |
| | | |
| | | |
| | | |
| | | |
| | | |
| | | |
| | | |
| | | |

## 6.6   Review

You are now well on your way to completing the foundation work for your Contentment Project.

Contentment project

| Chapter | Section | Progress |
|---|---|---|
| Who I am | | |
| | My history | ✓ |
| | Strengths | ✓ |
| | Preferences | ✓ |
| | Dark side | ✓ |
| Values | | |
| | Time analysis | ✓ |
| | Decision analysis | ✓ |
| | Worry analysis | ✓ |
| | Influences | ✓ |
| | Values statements | ✓ |
| Purpose | | |
| | Identifying Themes | ✓ |
| | Identifying Aspects | ✓ |
| | Action matrix | ✓ |
| | Objectives and plans | ✓ |
| Relationships | | |
| | Number of relationships | ✓ |
| | Groups of relationships | ✓ |
| | Quality and depth | ✓ |
| | Information flow | ✓ |
| | Energy input | ✓ |
| | Nuts and Bolts | ✓ |
| Resources | | |
| | Resource identification | ✓ |
| | Review action plans | ✓ |
| Achievements | | |
| | | |
| | | |

# Chapter 7

# Achievement

## Sections in Chapter 7

# Chapter 7

# Achievement

## 7.1    Why is this chapter important?

### Positive mood and positive energy.

Working through your Contentment Project requires energy and perseverance. It can't be completed overnight, and the process requires you to keep up a process of thinking and reviewing progress, then constantly updating your action plans. To keep this going, you need to feel it is worthwhile, and you need to feel you are getting somewhere.

In the Purpose chapter, you may remember the positive comment that *"we gain satisfaction and positive feedback from making progress towards a goal, not just when we attain the final objective."* Very helpfully, the cycle of action planning that you have been encouraged to use builds in the weekly reviewing of progress against each action plan, and creates positive feedback for you. This isn't just useful as part of the planning process. It is absolutely essential if you are to maintain motivation and energy in your project.

Imagine a long car journey. If you have no information about your progress it seems to go on forever. If you have plotted landmarks along the way it is much easier to think, "that's the first section complete", then "that's past the half-way mark", and so on. It is easier to maintain a feeling of progress and to keep up both your morale and your passengers' good humour if you can create positive snippets of information about progress.

If you work-out in a gym, you will be familiar with the way that feedback about progress keeps you going. On the treadmill, you can set yourself a distance to complete, and as you see the distance clocking up towards your target you keep going – even beyond the point when you feel tired and inclined to stop. When you achieve the distance you planned, you can experience a satisfaction that is much more important to your mood than any feeling of tiredness.

Similarly in your Contentment Project, you will experience feelings of tiredness, and moments of inclination not to bother. You can improve your level of energy and your inclination to keep going by creating the positive feedback that you need. The weekly review where you tick off the items you have completed, and see the physical evidence of progress towards the overall objective, is your self-administered dose of motivation and energy.

## Learning as you progress

It really helps if you regard the Project as a learning experience rather than as something that you can plan and implement perfectly. It is absolutely normal to make mistakes. You may plan to do too much at first. You may plan too little and fail to stretch yourself enough. Some people try to conquer mountains in the first week, and don't quite make it. They need to learn about the realities of what they can manage. Other people don't push hard enough and don't create enough feeling of progress. They need to learn to set their targets a little higher.

You will learn about yourself as well as learning about the mechanics of the Contentment Project. Your action plans will challenge and encourage you to make changes in your life. Some will work well, but some will not. You need to keep an honest self-appraisal active in your mind, so that you can learn what is realistic for you, and what is never going to be a comfortable fit for you.

## The Guided Missile

For many of us it is a negative experience to receive corrective feedback. This is a real pity! Imagine how liberating it would be to react positively and gratefully to all the corrective comments that people might make to us. When someone points out that you are driving too fast, rather than being annoyed at their cheek imagine feeling grateful for the information that indicates their level of discomfort. When someone criticises your choice of clothes, imagine gratefully filing away the useful data! When someone complains about your cooking, imagine being able to calmly analyse the information and plan some positive improvement!

Most of us don't find that our natural response. To help you move a little in that direction take comfort from the analogy of the guided missile. Essential to the accurate performance of a guided missile is the continual stream of little corrections it receives. It doesn't set off and unerringly hit the target. It receives second-by-second corrections from its guidance system. Put a human being in place of the machinery, and you introduce the risk of the human reacting huffily to the corrections. Try to think of yourself as the guided missile and take the feedback you can grab as valuable data to help your progress rather than as a threat to your happiness!

## 7.2 Perspective in achievement

Later in the chapter you will find some guidance on suggested frequency and detail of review of your achievements. A thought to keep in mind is the irrationality that we can display, and the extent to which this can be useful!

It may seem crazy, but you will probably find that little successes are just as valuable a boost to your morale as big successes. This is the useful aspect of our irrationality. When you create a task list, you create a potential for positive feedback. Each task you can tick off gives a positive boost to your morale and to your energy. It makes it easier to contemplate more progress tomorrow.

The suggested time-scale of reviews later in the chapter will encourage you to have a cycle where you have daily and weekly reviews of the achievable tasks, and monthly and even yearly reviews of the big picture. Don't underestimate the importance of either. They are both essential parts of the process. The little review of yesterday's task achievement is an essential building block for the more holistic review. It is a bonus that we are able to extract such disproportionate pleasure and satisfaction from small successes.

## 7.3 Activity plan reviews

Think of daily and weekly cycles for this basic level of activity. Depending on how you organise yourself, and on the nature of the task you set yourself, you will need to adjust the frequency of review to what works for you. You may find that this week you can romp through a series of achievements, and daily reviews are both necessary and rewarding. Next week you may find that other demands leave you with only a small amount of progress and you can review at the end of the week.

Take Jack's example of his action plan, where he started off with just two items in this particular Objective, and added a third when he thought about resources:

| Theme | Attention to family | | Objective: | I will have achieved a balance in my work-life that allows me to be a successful and hard worker while giving time and attention to my family.  I will no longer feel guilty about time allocation, and my family will be positive about my work and my time management. |
|---|---|---|---|---|
| Aspect | Work-life | | | |
| | | | | |

| | Item | Tick |
|---|---|---|
| Action: | Stop work by 6:00 pm on Friday | |
| | Check conference dates against family events | |
| | Explain Friday 6:00 pm plan to Trish and John and agree how we do it. | |
| | | |
| | | |
| | | |
| | | |
| | | |
| | | |
| | | |

Jack can probably make progress right away on the second task – checking conference dates against family events.  What he finds may lead to some further action plans, but at least he can probably tick that off within the first day.  Explaining his plan to Trish and John may take longer as he will need to find the opportune time to do this, but if he is going to achieve Friday's goal, he needs to get it done before then.  So you can imagine Jack reviewing this plan on a daily basis, and at the end of the week hopefully ticking off the success of leaving the office on time.  He might then need to create a new recurring task to make sure this isn't a one-off, but he has the potential for creating some achievement over the first week of his action plan, so it is worthwhile reviewing it frequently.

Allocate yourself time for these reviews.  I find that even 5-minutes of concentration in the morning can be enough to remind me of the immediate tasks and tick off the completed tasks.  Once a week you will need more time as you will be checking more thoughtfully what extra tasks you need to add, and what progress you are making towards your overall objectives.

## 7.4    Reviewing Objectives

Think about reviewing progress against the Objectives you have set on a monthly basis, and reviewing whether they are the right objectives on at least 6-monthly or possibly an annual basis.

If you have followed the suggested format, you will have between 6 and 12 active Objectives.  Chapter 8 will give some hints about how you can use a support group to help with this process, but for now we will assume you are working alone.  On a monthly basis, organise for yourself a location that suits you for concentrated thinking, and set aside a period of 1 – 2 hours to ask yourself,

- How am I doing against this Objective – what progress have I made?
- What Action Plans have I successfully completed?
- Do I need to add further Action Plans?
- What am I learning about myself in working on this Objective?

Make notes on the Objective sheets – or on the computer version you are using.   Make sure that you have sufficient peace and quiet to reflect thoroughly on each of the Objectives, and celebrate mentally the progress you are making.

You should emerge from one of these sessions energised, positive, and clutching an updated set of Objectives and Action Plans!   This is one of the key building blocks in your Contentment Project, and the satisfaction you can feel from making progress will help create the feeling of contentment that you are looking for.

## 7.5    Reviewing Aspects and Themes

Plan to review this overall chart only on an annual basis.  It is a very important project overview document, and it should be stable and long-lasting.  It reflects a very concise distillation of the thinking you have done about yourself, your nature, your values, your purpose, and the realities of the life within which you have to make sense of it all.

Once again you may find that the suggestions in Chapter 8 about use of a group will help with this very challenging process.  However if you are working alone, you can organise yourself so that this is a real landmark, rather than a non-event in the margins of your life.

If time and money allow, you may find you like to treat yourself to a "retreat" for the purposes of this review.  A quiet cottage looking over the sea will suit some of you.  I like to use my own study, but to choose a time when I can work undisturbed and out of the normal routine.

### Annual Review - Step 1 – back to basics

As groundwork you really need to go back to basics, so a good starting point is to re-read some of the review documents that you produced at the outset of the Project.

The key items to look back over are:

- Chapter 2 – Summary of Strengths – especially the "Action" column
- Same chapter – History – especially the "What can I learn?" column
- Same chapter – Flip side – especially the "Well?" column

- Chapter 3 – your statements at the end of the chapter "I want to live my life on the basis of……"
- Chapter 4 – your obituary.

When you have re-read these, you may want to add some notes on the basis of what you have learned about yourself in carrying the project this far. Some of the strengths you didn't realise you had may have shown themselves. Things you wondered could you do may now seem confidently achievable. Other strengths may have proved more elusive and need more work to become a reality. It will be surprising if you want to throw it all out. You are unlikely to find that the big themes are totally changed. Your Values statement and your obituary are likely to be just as good a reminder of your fundamental aspirations as they were a year before.

Make notes of any changes – things may seem even more important than they were originally. You may have made such progress that it is time to change where you put effort in your Action Plans.

## Annual Review - Step 2 - Themes and aspects

Having reviewed and reflected on that core material, go back to the Themes and Aspects you identified at the outset. This is a good opportunity for a strategic view of where you need to put energy and effort.

Jack's original chart looked like this: (next page)

| Aspect | Theme | | | | | | | |
| --- | --- | --- | --- | --- | --- | --- | --- | --- |
| | Attention to family | Community comtribution | Integrity | Friendship | Innovation | People rather than things | Relaxed and intuitive vs cold and logical | Health |
| Family life | | | | | | ✓ | ✓ | |
| Work life | ✓ | | ✓ | | ✓ | | ✓ | |
| Friends | | | | ✓ | | | | |
| Spare time | ✓ | ✓ | | ✓ | | | | ✓ |
| Holidays | | | | | ✓ | | | |

This key chart led Jack to the 12 Objectives that he set himself last year. The combination of reviewing his progress on each of the Objectives along with revisiting the worksheets listed above, allows Jack to think again about which of the Themes really need attention in the coming year.

Jack has made great progress in managing his work life in order to allow the more obvious attention to family that he planned. However he knows that this is something that needs to stay on his agenda – otherwise work will take over again.

When Jack reviews each of the items he is pleased to be able to see progress in most of them. But he hasn't made progress on the Community Contribution that he planned, and he is ever more aware that Health is a precious bonus that needs more work. So his overall chart maybe can be amended to look like this:

| Aspect | Theme | | | | | | | |
|---|---|---|---|---|---|---|---|---|
| | Attention to family | Community comtribution | Integrity | Friendship | Innovation | People rather than things | Relaxed and intuitive vs cold and logical | Health |
| Family life | | | | | | ✓ | | |
| Work life | ✓ | | ✓ | | ✓ | | ✓ | |
| Friends | | | | ✓ | | | | ✓ |
| Spare time | ✓ | ✓✓ | | | | | | ✓ |
| Holidays | | | | | | | | |

Jack has been able to adjust his chart as he is happy that the progress on being less cold and logical in the family context has been achieved. He is happy that they have created a new pattern for holidays, and that target can be reassigned. He indicates the emphasis he wants to put on the Community Contribution, this having been a more difficult objective than any other to progress. He also shifts some emphasis so that he will be pushing himself to increase the emphasis on Health, but constructively building in some new context for doing that with his friends. Overall he is able to drop 3 of the previous Objective sheets he had used, one needs to be re-thought so that he really can make progress on his Community Contribution, and he needs a new Objective sheet relating to Friends and Health.

## 7.6 Updating Objectives

Back to the hard work again.  You will now need to create the revised set of Objective and Task sheets for the coming year.  Start with clean sheets even for those that are continuing from last year, and create any new sheets that are needed.  The following pages provide space for 6 once again.  Photocopy as necessary.

| Theme | | Objective: | |
|---|---|---|---|
| Aspect | | | |

| Action: | Item | Tick |
|---|---|---|
| | | |
| | | |
| | | |
| | | |
| | | |
| | | |
| | | |
| | | |
| | | |
| | | |
| | | |

| Theme | | Objective: | |
|---|---|---|---|
| Aspect | | | |

| Action: | Item | Tick |
|---|---|---|
| | | |
| | | |
| | | |
| | | |
| | | |
| | | |
| | | |
| | | |
| | | |
| | | |
| | | |

| Theme | | Objective: | |
|---|---|---|---|
| Aspect | | | |

| Action: | Item | Tick |
|---|---|---|
| | | |
| | | |
| | | |
| | | |
| | | |
| | | |
| | | |
| | | |
| | | |
| | | |
| | | |

| Theme | | Objective: | |
|---|---|---|---|
| Aspect | | | |

| Action: | Item | Tick |
|---|---|---|
| | | |
| | | |
| | | |
| | | |
| | | |
| | | |
| | | |
| | | |
| | | |
| | | |

| Theme | | Objective: | |
|---|---|---|---|
| Aspect | | | |

| Action: | Item | Tick |
|---|---|---|
| | | |
| | | |
| | | |
| | | |
| | | |
| | | |
| | | |
| | | |
| | | |
| | | |

| Theme | | Objective: | |
|---|---|---|---|
| Aspect | | | |

| Action: | Item | Tick |
|---|---|---|
| | | |
| | | |
| | | |
| | | |
| | | |
| | | |
| | | |
| | | |
| | | |
| | | |

## 7.7    Keeping track of the Project

Also on an annual basis you will want to keep track of the impact of all of this on your life and on your contentment.  This is not as simple as taking your blood pressure or your temperature!  Feelings of Contentment are by nature subjective and elusive, but we can try to keep track of the components and create a useful picture of progress.

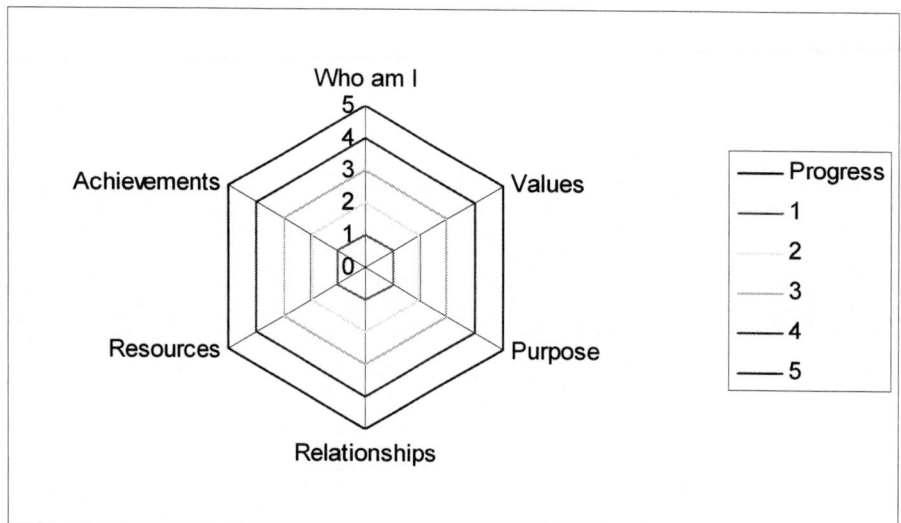

1 = Just started

2 = Some progress

3 = Half-way there

4 = Very significant progress

5 = Satisfied with work completed

If you think back over each of these sections of the book, you may be able to identify the extent to which you have satisfied yourself with the progress you have made.  If you are completely satisfied that you have made full use of the exercises in that section, and that you have honestly completed the self-analysis, you can award yourself a score of 5.  If you have not yet started work on the section award yourself a 0!  You may end up with a chart that looks like this, and a very graphic way of reminding yourself of the work you need to do:

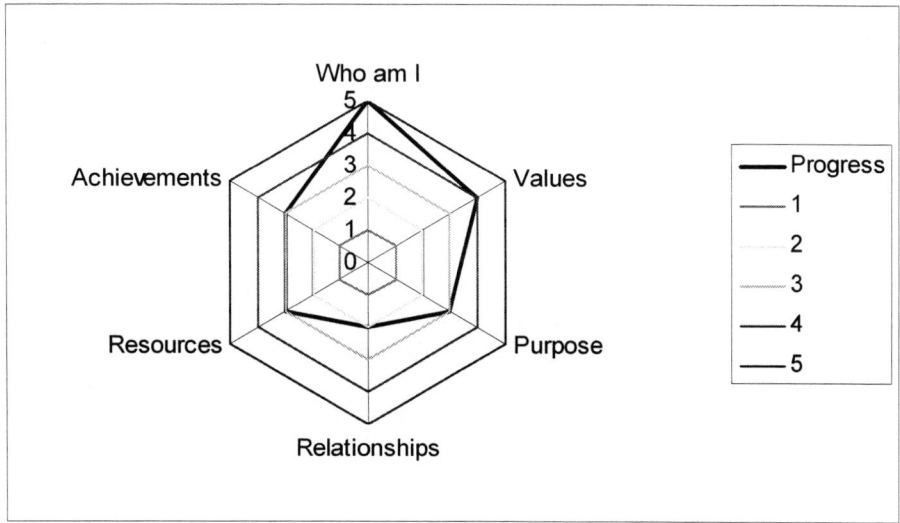

In this example, I have done a really good job on the "Who am I " section, and have made good progress on my Values.  However I still have work to do on the others, especially the Relationships section, where I have made least progress.

If you create a chart like this it really speeds up your review process – you can see at a glance where you are.  This is extremely useful if you use a group and want to share information.

## 7.8  Summary

This chapter has dealt with the way in which keeping track of your achievement is essential for your motivation; your energy; your learning; and for its contribution to your Contentment.

It has suggested a daily, weekly and longer-term cycle of reviews that you can use to keep track not only of the short-term action plans, but also of the overall Contentment Project.

The timing of your review processes will be highly individual, but an outline might be as follows:

|  | Task list | Objectives (progress) | Resources | Themes and Aspects | Overall progress (revise Objectives) |
|---|---|---|---|---|---|
| Daily | ✓ | | | | |
| Weekly | ✓ | | | | |
| Monthly | | ✓ | | | |
| Quarterly | | ✓ | ✓ | | |
| Yearly | | | | ✓ | ✓ |

# Chapter 8

# Rolling on

**Sections in Chapter 8**

# Chapter 8

# Rolling on

## 8.1   Review

This book has asked you to do a lot of structured thinking and reviewing of yourself and your life.  As you have worked your way through the exercises, you have been asking yourself fundamental questions about who you are, what values you hold, what purpose there is to your life.

These are not questions that allow you to come up with one quick and neat answer.  Some of us find that part of our human nature is to experience recurring disquiet, and an urge to question and to change.  These are not feelings and thoughts to be feared.  They are natural and are part of what keeps us alert and drives our development.  However we need a firm foundation so that we can maintain our balance and self-confidence while facing serious questions about our nature and our life.

This book has taken you through a process that will have allowed you to check the extent to which you put into practice the "habits" that are demonstrated by the most contented people.

You should now be able to:

- Think and speak clearly and honestly about who you are – your strengths, weaknesses and preferences;
- Describe and use your Values Statements – describing what is important to you and the principles that guide your decisions;
- Make use of the Objectives and Action Plans you have established – creating a feeling of purpose and motivation;

- Develop, value and enjoy the relationships you have with other people;
- List and use the resources that are available to you – whether personal, physical, or in other people;
- List and celebrate your progress and your achievements in turning your objectives and action plans into reality.

## 8.2  Alone or with help?

If you have worked your way through the exercises on your own you may have wondered how much of a difference it would make to share the thoughts with someone else.  If you have a partner, you probably have been sharing with them.  If your style and preference is to work through these thoughts on your own, then that is what you have probably done.  You may find it useful to reflect on the "Who am I" section again to check the extent to which the preferences you identified there are a good fit with the way that you have dealt with the question of solo or shared working.  The scoring you gave yourself in the Social and Action sections will be very relevant.  If you feel it would be beneficial to share the thoughts, then you need to plan and organise yourself to do that.  If you feel happy working on your own - don't worry.  That is perfectly reasonable.  Working in the way that suits your preferences is all you are asked to do.

## 8.3  Shared working with friend or partner

You will find that the guidelines in the Relationships chapter on the Nuts and Bolts of getting together are very relevant to this section.  You should try to avoid misunderstandings and unhelpful exchanges by making sure that you both are clear  about what you are doing, and by managing things in such a way that you enhance the opportunities you have to meet, rather than making them a challenge.

This can be a really helpful process – enhancing your analysis of your own strengths and preferences – as well as providing some extra motivation and drive to progress with your Project.  However people can have very different experiences of sharing.

> *Jack started work on his Contentment Project with great enthusiasm.  He was convinced that he could benefit enormously from the process, and his "Who am I" analysis fired his imagination as he had never before devoted structured time to such thoughts.  As he worked through his "Values" he decided to share the work with his wife.  She was not tuned in to the process, was busy with other issues and reacted negatively to the whole idea.*
>
> *On reflection he realised that he had handled things badly. He had not thought about the explanations that would help his wife tune in to the subject, and had not chosen the time sensitively.  As a result he had to take time to approach the whole issue again a few weeks later, and eventually made some progress with the sharing. However he realised afterwards that he could have helped things go smoothly if he had used a friend as his initial speaking-partner.  His wife was much more inclined to be helpful when she had experienced some of the progress Jack made in his work/life balance.*

Try to use this checklist in preparing to share with a partner or close friend:

- Have I explained the context – what I'm trying to do?
- Is the time right?

- Is the other person preoccupied with other pressing issues?
- Is the other person able to tune in to the same level of thinking now? (This is not an implied criticism!  If I am up to my eyes with a leaking pipe, an expensive car repair, and a looming deadline for some work, I am unlikely to be able to think helpfully if my wife wants to talk philosophy or politics!)
- What am I looking for – Support?  Challenge?  Agreement?  Can I cope with challenge?

## 8.4 Group activity

It can be really helpful to make use of a "support and challenge" group to help you with the Contentment Project.  If you think that you would work better that way, this section is for you.  If you prefer to work alone – don't worry.

## Suggestions for setting up a group to work together

Try to identify at least two and at most four other people who can work with you.  Ideally they should be:

- Naturally interested in their own contentment project
- Not too closely involved in any of your problem areas of life
- Unthreatened by open discussion of innermost thoughts and feelings
- Trustworthy and confidential
- With no "agenda" relating to what they want you to do.

If you can identify potential group members, float the idea and let them read some sample parts of the book to test their reaction. If they are tempted by the ideas then you will have a positive and useful group.

## 8.5 Agenda for group work

It makes sense to work through the book in the order in which it is presented. You might want to have a couple of introductory meetings where you use the Introductory chapter as a basis for discussion of what you all want to get from the process, and to share ideas about ground-rules.

The following is a possible format:

| Meeting | Theme | Agenda | Action for next time |
|---------|-------|--------|---------------------|
| 1 | Introductions and expectations | • What we want out of this<br>• Ground-rules (confidentiality, ability to challenge, logistics) | Read Intro |
| 2<br>(one week later) | Project Planning | • Reactions to Introduction<br>• Clarification of expectations<br>• Meeting dates/times | Read "Who am I" and complete History line |
| 3<br>(two weeks later) | Who am I | • Compare reactions<br>• Share History lines<br>• Discuss learning | Complete Strengths questionnaires |
| 4<br>(two weeks later) | Who am I | • Review of strengths (one person at a time)<br>• Feedback (confirmation or challenge)<br>• Confirmation of key learning for each person | Complete Preferences questionnaires |
| 5<br>(two weeks later) | Who am I | • Review of preferences (one person at a time)<br>• Feedback (confirmation, challenge, evidence) | Complete Dark side and Flip side exercises |

| Meeting | Theme | Agenda | Action for next time |
|---|---|---|---|
| 6 – 12 onwards | Work your way as above through the subject areas | Try to be structured and organised in the time allocated to each person for review of the work-sheets. This format will take you through the First 4 Chapters – the point where you have identified Objectives and associated Action plans | Complete the exercises in Chapters 3 and 4, agreeing clearly each time what will be done for next session. |
| 13 (approx) | Relationships plus action points | • Quick review of progress on agreed action points<br><br>• Next action points<br><br>• Review of Relationship questionnaires<br><br>• Learning from the data<br><br>• Action? | Read and complete the Resources section. |
| 14 (approx) | Resources plus action points | • Quick review of progress on agreed action points<br><br>• Next action points<br><br>• Review of Resource questionnaires<br><br>• Learning from the data<br><br>• Additions and amendments to Action points? | Read Achievement chapter |

| Meeting | Theme | Agenda | Action for next time |
|---------|-------|--------|----------------------|
| 15 (approx) | Rolling on | • Review of progress on action points<br>• Discussion of Achievement chapter<br>• Discussion and agreement on pattern of further meetings<br>• Action plans | |
| 20 (approx) | Annual review of person (a) | • Rethink of Themes and Aspects<br>• Re-jig of key areas<br>• Review of Objectives<br>• Review of progress on action plans<br>• Summary of "How am I" – progress on Contentment Project? | |
| 21 (approx) | Annual review of person (b) | • As above | |
| 22 (approx) | Annual review of person (c) | • As above | |
| 23 | Where next | • Group review of whole process<br>• Do we continue?<br>• Celebrate success<br>• Agree closure/or action | |

## 8.6    Winding up and summing up

Many people will want to change their mode of using the material after one complete cycle of the thinking, the action planning, and the achievement. Some of the habits and approaches will have become normal and intrinsic ways of operating and thinking, so the explicit exercises may become less important.  It may become a useful monthly check to use some of the Themes, Aspects and Objectives to do a short-hand review of life, rather than feeling bound by the mechanisms.

It is important to avoid empty repetition – better to have a break and come back 6 months later to review how things are going, than to feel obliged to keep to a routine.  This is particularly important for a group. Better by far to end on a high note of completion of a cycle of the book rather than allowing motivation and attendance to gradually dwindle.

Whatever onward process you choose, you will go forward with a greater level of contentment in your life having used the exercises and the thought process of the book.  Contentment is not an unbroken state of untroubled bliss!  It is a *"state of happiness and contentment in life, which is more long-lasting and pervasive than a reaction or temporary mood, and is more firmly based and conscious than a simple cheerful disposition."*

I hope that this book has helped you find that firmer base for your contentment, so that you have the strength and resilience to deal with the inevitable ups and downs that all of us encounter.